THE
Chemotherapy &
Radiation Therapy
SURVIVAL GUIDE

JUDITH McKAY, R.N., O.C.N.
NANCEE HIRANO, R.N., M.S., A.O.C.N.

NEW HARBINGER PUBLICATIONS, INC.

Publisher's Note

This publication is designed to provide accurate and authoritative information in regard to the subject matter covered. It is sold with the understanding that the publisher is not engaged in rendering psychological, financial, legal, or other professional services. If expert assistance or counseling is needed, the services of a competent professional should be sought.

Drawings on pages 46, 47, 52, and 53 used with the permission of Abbott Laboratories and originally appeared in their booklet "Venous Access Device Occlusions." Drawings on pages 49 and 51 adapted from "Venous Access Device Occlusions" by SHELBY DESIGNS & ILLUSTRATES.

Distributed in Canada by Raincoast Books

Copyright © 1998 by Judith McKay, R.N., O.C.N. and Nancee Hirano R.N., M.S., A.O.C.N
New Harbinger Publications, Inc.
5674 Shattuck Avenue
Oakland, CA 94609

Cover design by SHELBY DESIGNS & ILLUSTRATES.
Edited by Carole Honeychurch
Text design by Michele Waters

Library of Congress Catalog Number: 97-69490
ISBN 1-57224-070-9

Printed in the United States of America on recycled paper.

New Harbinger Publications' Web site address: www.newharbinger.com

08   07   06

20   19   18   17   16

For my husband Matthew, and to the memory of my father, Benjamin Becker.

—J.Mc.

To my husband, Terence Shinsato, my parents, Yutaka and Taeko, and to Sammy; to the memory of my mother-in-law, Grace Shinsato.

—N.H.

Acknowledgments

We are grateful to the following people who've been extremely helpful in the development of this book. Michael Casssidy, M.D., Laurie Cardella, R.N., Marianne Caseri, R.N., Mary Bloom, R.N., Kate Tierney, R.N., M.S.N., and Inga Aksamit, R.N. reviewed the chapter "Bone Marrow and Stem-Cell Transplant" for clarity and accuracy.

Janet Lyle, Pharm.D., and Holly Schenck, R.N., gave us valuable feedback on several chapters. Mary Hoffman contributed to "Relaxation and Stress Reduction." Our colleagues, Tinrin Chew, R.D., Cathy Kyne, R.N., Joanne Rollins-Noyes, R.N., Christina Pulliam, R.N., Lori Gitter, R.N., and Martha Tracy, M.D., shared their expertise.

We appreciate Helen Crothers, M.S.W., and the Alta Bates Foundation, whose support for *The Chemotherapy Survival Guide* made the book available, free of charge, for all of the patients receiving treatment at the center.

We would also like to thank our patients who, by sharing their experiences with us, gave us a better understanding of how we could help others.

Contents

Introduction

A survival guide is a book of directions to help travelers cope with difficulties or unusual circumstances. It provides essential information, practical suggestions, and encouragement so that travelers can use their own resources and the resources in their environment to make it through the obstacles along the way.

Many people who are facing cancer therapy for the first time feel like they have been dropped behind enemy lines during a war. They don't know the language or the terrain and don't know what to expect or what is expected of them. The hospital or clinic environment and technical medical terminology are foreign. All of these circumstances add to the feeling of being lost in an alien world. A person recovering from the stress of recent cancer surgery may feel even more overwhelmed. And it may be difficult to get needed support if friends and family are busy dealing with their own fears and misconceptions about cancer and cancer-fighting treatments.

This book is meant to be a survival guide. It explains what chemotherapy and radiation therapy are, how they work, and how they may affect you. It contains simple and understandable answers for many of the questions you may have. Most importantly, it gives you practical suggestions about what you can do to help yourself while receiving treatment. These are the same hints and suggestions that nurses give their patients based on the nurses' experience and the experiences of the many people who have gone through these treatments.

Cancer-Fighting Treatments

Before chemotherapy or radiation therapy, the most common treatment for cancer was surgery. But if the cancer was in an area that couldn't be surgically removed, or if some cancer cells had spread to other areas of the body, no effective treatment was available. In those days, surgery tended to be more radical, often removing large areas of healthy tissue in an attempt to catch the few microscopic cancer cells that might have escaped from the original tumor.

One distinguishing characteristic of most cancer cells is their tendency to divide frequently—too frequently—in a way that is out of control. This tendency means that any drug or treatment that can damage cells in the dividing stage will have a far greater effect on cancer cells than most normal tissue.

Chemotherapy is the term used to identify the various drugs that fight cancer. These drugs travel throughout the body and are able to damage the rapidly dividing cells (like tumor cells) so they are not able to continue to grow. It does this by interfering with the cell's life cycle at different stages. Many of the side effects of chemotherapy are caused by the chemotherapy's effect on normal cells that are also dividing frequently, such as the cells of the digestive tract or the bone marrow where blood cells are produced.

The first chemical therapy treatments used this principle to kill frequently dividing cells in the blood (leukemia) and the lymph system (lymphoma). Since then, more than fifty cancer-fighting drugs have been developed using this same approach. Researchers continue to explore how these drugs can be used alone and in combination with other drugs to make this form of treatment even more effective.

Radiation therapy is the term used to identify the cancer-fighting treatment that uses radiation energy (produced by X rays and other radioactive sources) to kill cancer cells. Radiation interacts with the atoms and molecules in the cell and either kills the cell or damages it so it cannot reproduce. Cells that are dividing frequently, such as tumor cells, are generally more sensitive to the effects of radiation. Radiation was first used to treat skin cancer, but today, high-energy radiation and modern methods can deliver treatment to tumors that may lie deep within the body as well. Unlike chemotherapy, radiation does not affect cells throughout the body, but only the area exposed to the radiation. Many of the side effects of radiation therapy are associated with radiation's effect on normal tissue that may also be exposed to radiation during the treatments.

Modern chemotherapy and radiation therapy are powerful and in many cases highly effective weapons in the fight against cancer. For some kinds of cancer that are particularly vulnerable to the effects of radiation therapy, it may be the only treatment necessary. For other kinds of cancer, chemotherapy alone is effective to kill cancer cells, prevent the spread of the disease, and significantly improve the chances for recovery. Many people receive both chemotherapy and radiation therapy along with other forms of treatment such as surgery or hormonal therapy. Sometimes chemotherapy or radiation therapy are recommended even when all measurable signs of cancer are gone. This is just to make sure that any possible spread of cancer cells—even on a microscopic level—is eliminated.

What This Book Offers

Most people know very little about what to expect when they are getting chemotherapy or radiation therapy. They may be aware of some potential side effects such as nausea or hair loss, but they don't know whether these reactions will happen to them or what, if anything, they can do about them.

The purpose of this book is to answer many of your questions about cancer, chemotherapy, and radiation therapy. Moreover, it offers guidance for how you can help yourself during your treatment. What does radiation therapy feel like? How is chemotherapy given? What should you do before, during, and after each treatment? What can you expect at home? Why do you need so many blood tests? What do the tests show about how your body is reacting to the treatments?

You do not need to read this book from beginning to end—you can turn to any chapter for information and suggestions about the specific issue that concerns you.

The first two chapters explain the basic facts about chemotherapy and radiation therapy—how each works to kill cancer cells, the side effects that you can expect, and the reason these side effects may occur. Chapter 3 ("Understanding Blood Tests") explains the reasons for and significance of the many blood tests you may need during your treatment. Chemotherapy is often given into your vein (a technique referred to as "intravenous" or "IV"). Chapter 4 provides information about how to cope with "The IV Experience"—problems that may arise as well as coping strategies to help you get through it.

At the heart of the guide are chapters describing the different side effects that might occur because of the way chemotherapy and radiation therapy affect healthy cells. At the beginning of each of these chapters is a review of why the chemotherapy or radiation therapy can cause that specific side effect, followed by many suggestions of what you can do to prevent, minimize, or manage the side effect. Accompanying these coping chapters is a chapter focusing on how to maintain good nutrition even when you are experiencing temporary changes in your appetite or digestion.

Bone marrow or peripheral stem-cell transplants are treatment options for some people when higher than standard doses of cancer-fighting therapy may be needed. Chapter 11 ("Bone Marrow and Stem-Cell Transplant") explains how these procedures are done, the expected side effects of the treatments, and ways of coping with them.

Chapter 12 ("Mind and Body") was written by a psychiatrist with many years of experience counseling patients and families who are dealing with the stress of cancer treatments. Chapter 13 provides relaxation and stress-reduction techniques to lower your anxiety, and Chapter 14 contains scripts you can use to make your own audio tape for healing visualizations. Finally, if you are having trouble distinguishing between the generic and brand names of some medications, there is a drug appendix in the back of the book to assist you.

What This Book Can't Do

This book does not include information about the individual chemotherapy drugs or combinations of drugs used to treat specific kinds of cancer. Your doctor will prescribe the chemotherapy medications and dosages based on the kind of cancer you have, its location, and its cellular characteristics, as well as your age, physical condition, and how well you are tolerating the treatment. Because there are so many different drugs, dosages, and combinations that are now used to fight cancer, this book doesn't include descriptions of each drug. Your doctor or nurse will provide you with that information and review the potential side effects with you.

This book is not a substitute for calling the doctor if you have a problem. There are many things about your specific treatment or symptoms that may need the physician's immediate attention. What you may consider to be just a little cough or a cold may require antibiotics or lab tests when you are taking chemotherapy or radiation therapy. An ache or swelling or rash can also be more significant during cancer-fighting therapy. So don't be shy about calling with a problem, symptom, or question. Keep in mind that you will probably develop a closer connection with your oncologist (the specialist in cancer care) and the nurses in the clinic than you may have had with health care providers in the past.

Cancer therapy is stressful, both physically and emotionally. But if you know what to expect, you will feel less overwhelmed. If you understand what problems may arise and what you can do to feel better, you will feel more empowered. If you are armed with practical suggestions and a coping plan to deal with problems, you can feel more in control. This survival guide can help make the journey easier by providing the information and sources of support you need to face the challenge and make it through.

1

What Is Chemotherapy?

In order to understand how chemotherapy will help you, you first must understand how cancer cells are different from normal cells. You need to understand how cancer cells grow and how their growth can be stopped.

A Primer on Cell Life

All living things are made up of cells, and each cell has a life of its own. Cells are the basic building blocks of life. When you look at a one-cell organism (like the amoeba you may have seen under the microscope in biology class), you can identify different cell structures that keep the cell working, dividing, and surviving. A *cell wall* surrounds the cell and separates it from its environment and determines what goes in and what goes out. Within the cell is a very important structure called the *nucleus*, the cell's command center. The nucleus directs and controls all of a cell's functions and determines how and when it divides. Within the nucleus is the *DNA*, which is like a master computer program for that cell.

When the cell divides, it splits into two identical pieces. First, the DNA splits in half and duplicates itself, so that each half will have a complete and identical DNA program for that cell. Then the cell membrane and all the other structures divide. Each new daughter cell is exactly like the original parent cell, with identical cell parts, nucleus, and DNA information.

Complex life forms like ourselves are made up of millions of cells. Groups of cells perform different specialized functions to keep the whole system working well. Some are part of the heart muscle and have the ability to contract. Other cells are part of the digestive system and secrete enzymes or absorb nutrients. Some are part of the liver and function to filter the blood and store energy. But all cells work together to keep the big system, the human body, alive and well in its environment. All cells are living, growing, and at times dividing in a specific and controlled way based on a program contained in the DNA.

Characteristics of Normal Cells

Normal cells grow in a limited space and stay within their boundaries. Bone cells don't grow into the muscles that surround them; stomach cells don't grow into the space that the pancreas occupies (even though they lie right next to each other).

Normal cells divide at a set and controlled rate, depending on their function, their life span, and the information contained in their DNA. Some cells have a short life span and divide frequently. For example, the life span for some white blood cells is only seventy-two hours. The life span for a cell in your intestines is only two weeks. Other cells have a longer life span. The average red blood cell will live three to four months.

Some cells live as long as you do, dividing only to replace themselves if there has been an injury. For instance, if an adult breaks his arm, the bone cells are turned on to repair the damage. Once the injury heals, then bone cells in an adult divide very rarely. In fact, there are some cells which never divide again once they have grown to adult size. Brain cells do not divide and replace themselves even when damaged. The rate that normal cells divide is specific to each group and strictly controlled by their DNA program. This program is different for each type of cell.

Normal cells have a tendency to stick together so that cells do not break off and float away, even though the blood flows by each and every cell. If a normal cell were to break off into the blood and lodge elsewhere in the body, it would soon die. Normal cells are well *differentiated*, meaning that a pathologist can easily identify what kind of cell it is, what it does, and where it comes from. Liver cells look different than bladder cells, bone cells are quite distinct from brain cells. Cells with different functions vary as to size, shape, and diameter of the nucleus.

How Cells Are Nourished

Every one of the body's cells is washed continuously with blood. The blood carries oxygen from the lungs and nutrients from the digestive system. The blood is pumped by the heart through big arteries, then smaller and smaller vessels, until the blood reaches each and every cell, delivering oxygen and energy. Then, the blood picks up waste products that are produced by the cells and carries them to the filtering and cleansing organs (kidneys, liver, lungs) to be recycled or eliminated by the body. Every time you exhale, you get rid of some of the waste products (carbon dioxide) of cell activity. And when you urinate, you are eliminating waste products filtered out by your kidneys. Your blood is really a kind of transport system that trucks in life-sustaining supplies and then hauls off the debris.

How Cells Are Protected

The immune system provides mobile defenses for the body, sending out white blood cells (you might call them "soldier cells") that seek and destroy bacteria and viruses. White blood cells are mixed in the blood and wash along with it past every cell. They gather at the site of infections, surrounding and killing bacteria and viruses, and eventually migrate by way of lymph ducts to the lymph glands (or lymph nodes).

Lymph nodes are like a cluster of grapes, and act as filtering stations at various locations in your body. Each cluster of nodes receives *lymphocytes* (one type of white blood cell) that have washed past a certain organ. The lymph nodes are the places where the bacteria, worn-out lymphocytes, and debris are filtered and destroyed. You aren't usually aware of your lymph nodes unless they are swollen and tender from fighting infection. For example, you might feel swollen lymph nodes in your neck or under your jaw from a sore throat or an infected tooth. You might feel lymph nodes in your groin from a pelvic infection or in your armpit from an infection in your hand. Doctors know where to find the particular cluster of lymph nodes that filter each organ. They know where to feel for signs of infection and which lymph nodes to examine under the microscope when looking for cancer cells.

Characteristics of Cancer Cells

Cancer begins as a mutation or change in the DNA of a single normal cell in any part of the body. Once this change takes place, the set of instructions in the DNA is changed and the cell no longer acts like it normally does. Often a mutation or change results in a cell so damaged that it cannot survive or it fails to divide successfully. But if it does survive and divide, that mutated cell may look and act very differently from the cells around it.

Cancer cells look different. They may have a different size or shape or have larger or smaller nuclei. They may not fit together in an orderly, predictable arrangement of cells. They may not be able to do the job that they were designed to do.

Cancer cells often ignore the normal rate of cell division because they lack a growth-control mechanism. They may divide very rapidly, crowding, pushing, or blocking other organs and preventing them from doing their jobs. Because they don't stay within their boundaries, but instead, grow into surrounding organs, they are said to be *invasive.* Cancer cells frequently appear immature because they may divide several times before they are fully grown. They are also more likely to mutate again.

Whereas normal cells have a tendency to stick together, cancer cells are more likely to detach from the original location and move, via the bloodstream, to other areas of the body. They are also more likely to travel by way of the lymph system to the lymph nodes downstream and then to other organ systems. Most of these detached cells are usually destroyed by the body's defense system or filtered and eliminated like bacteria and other cell debris. But if the detached cancer cells do survive, they may produce a new growth at a different site or damage other organs as well.

Some Terms You Should Know

Hyperplasia is an increase in the number of cells at a particular site. It's a normal response to healing a broken bone or a surgical incision. It means that the cells are growing and dividing more quickly until the bone or scar is healed, when growth can slow down to its usual pace. The cells grow in an orderly, regular way and are easily identifiable (well differentiated). They look and act like normal cells.

Dysplasia is an overgrowth of cells that do not have the arrangement or function of normal cells. *Neoplasia* means new growth and describes the growth of cells beyond their normal boundaries. These new cells may be cancerous (*malignant*) or noncancerous (*benign*). Noncancerous overgrowth is well differentiated, and the cells look similar to other normal cells of the same organ. Such a growth usually divides slowly and is often encased in a limited area. It doesn't invade the tissue around it, nor will it travel to any other parts of the body. A benign cyst is an example of a noncancerous neoplasia.

A malignant tumor is an overgrowth of cells that often looks very dissimilar to normal cells in that organ. The cells may appear immature, divide quickly, and grow in a less orderly way. They may not be enclosed in a limited area and can invade the surrounding tissue. They can also detach from the tumor into the lymph system or the blood system and migrate to distant parts of the body. Some may survive and begin dividing in this new region.

When a little bit of tumor is removed and examined under a microscope, this procedure is called a *biopsy*. A pathologist will look at a few cells from the tumor to see how they compare to normal cells of that organ, and can determine whether the tumor has invaded surrounding tissue. By looking at nearby lymph glands, the pathologist can see if parts of the tumor have detached and are growing there.

Cancerous cells that have detached and traveled by the blood or lymph system usually cannot survive the blood pressure or the body's defense systems. Occasionally, however, they may lodge in an area where the blood pressure is low and blood moves slowly. The cancerous cells may grow there. This spread of cancer cells to another distant organ site is called *metastasis*.

From the very beginning, a doctor wants to know everything possible about the cancer. He or she gets that information with the help of many tests, including a biopsy, X rays, scans, and blood tests. Sometimes even the DNA of the cancerous cell is examined. This information-gathering process is called *staging*.

The results of all the tests will determine what kind of treatment you need.

Some cancerous cells produce substances that can be measured by a simple blood test. These substances are called *tumor markers* because they can indicate the presence of cancer cells, even if the cells cannot be seen. Not all cancers produce tumor markers. But if your cancer cells produce a tumor marker and the tumor marker measures higher than normal, it may indicate an increase in cancer cells. When the tumor marker drops, it usually indicates that there are fewer of these cells and that the tumor is responding to treatment. The doctor uses the tumor marker as important information in treatment decisions.

Treatment

Surgery

This is the oldest method of treating cancer, and sometimes it is the only treatment necessary. This is more likely to be true if the cancer is small, contained, and has not spread to adjacent tissue or spread through the lymph system or the blood system. At the time of surgery, the tumor is removed along with some of the healthy surrounding tissue. Often lymph nodes from adjacent areas are also removed so that the pathologist can see if they have some cancerous cells growing in them.

If the cancer has spread, or if it is an aggressive type of cancer with a high likelihood of spreading to other organs, additional anticancer treatments may be recommended. In many cases, these additional treatments are recommended even if the original cancer is small, contained, and shows no sign of spreading to other areas.

Radiation

This treatment uses high-energy particles that can penetrate through your body. Special machines generate and direct these particles to a specific place for a specific amount of time. A specialist (the radiation oncologist) calculates the exact area, amount, and frequency of radiation treatments based on the kind of tumor, location, biopsies, and so on. Normal tissues are shielded, and the radiation beam is precisely aimed at the tumor so it gets a high dose of radiation and the normal tissue does not. Cells that are dividing frequently, like cancer cells, are especially sensitive to radiation. When these high-energy particles are directed at a tumor site, they damage or destroy these cells. Radiation damages the cell's DNA, cell membranes, and other cell structures.

Radiation may be the only treatment necessary if the cancer cells are very sensitive to its effects and there is no sign that the cancer has spread. Radiation treatment may be given before surgery to shrink a tumor so it can more easily be removed. Or, it may be given along with or following chemotherapy because some of the chemotherapy medicines make cancer cells more sensitive to the effects of radiation. Radiation may be suggested after surgery even if there are no detectable cancer cells in the lymph or surrounding tissue just to make sure no cells have escaped.

Chapter 2 ("What Is Radiation Therapy?") has a full explanation of this form of treatment, the side effects, and many self-help suggestions.

Chemotherapy

The medicines used to treat cancer include a large group of different drugs. Some, like hormones and steroids, have familiar uses other than the treatment of cancer. But any drug or combination of drugs that kills, slows down, or damages cancer cells can be considered chemotherapy.

You are familiar with medicines that treat bacterial infection, such as antibiotics. Once they enter your bloodstream, these drugs usually have little effect on the rest of your body. It is the bacteria that are sensitive to and are killed by the antibiotics. But since cancer cells are not a foreign invader, but instead are damaged, mutated human cells, anticancer medicine has to work in a different way. It has to kill cancer cells without permanently damaging normal cells.

No current anticancer medicine attacks just cancer cells without affecting some normal cells. Since chemotherapy damages cancer cells that are rapidly dividing, those normal cells that are dividing rapidly are also affected by the drugs.

Some chemotherapy drugs interfere with the sequence of activities that a cell must go through to divide into two identical daughter cells. If the cell can't divide, then it will live out its life span and die. Drugs that act this way are called *cell cycle specific*. They prevent cancer cells from reproducing at a particular phase of the cell's life span.

Other chemotherapy drugs affect cancer cells in all phases of life. But because cancer cells are often more immature or fragile than normal cells, these drugs affect cancer cells far more than healthy cells. These medicines are called *cell cycle nonspecific* since they kill cancer cells at any time during the cell's life span without waiting for them to divide. These drugs are especially useful in killing cancer cells that are slow-growing.

Other drugs can make the environment less hospitable to cancer cells and thus slow them down. Hormones work this way. For instance, some breast cancer tumors grow faster in the presence of estrogen, and some prostate cancers grow faster in the presence of testosterone. Hormones that block estrogen or testosterone can discourage the growth of those cancer cells.

Combinations of Drugs

Years ago people were usually given one chemotherapy drug at a time. Now, with further research and the development of new drugs, doctors may recommend a combination of chemotherapy drugs. This combination of drugs can often be more effective at killing cancer cells than using one drug alone. Anticancer drugs with different modes of action and which produce different side effects are usually combined. For instance, you may be given a chemotherapy drug that kills the cancer cells while they are dividing, and you may also be given a chemotherapy drug which kills cells even when they are not dividing. You may also take a hormone which will change the environment of the cancer cells and discourage their growth.

Using a combination of drugs that work in different ways can make chemotherapy more deadly to cancer cells and less toxic to healthy cells. The specific drug or combination of drugs recommended, as well as the schedule of how frequently you get treatments, depends on a number of things—the kind of cancer, its location, and how quickly your healthy cells recover from the treatment.

Side Effects

You take medicine for some desired effect. Different medicines can lower blood pressure, relieve pain, kill bacteria, and so on. The effects are usually predictable and beneficial. But medicines often have other effects which may be predictable, but are not necessarily beneficial. Side effects are undesired consequences that inevitably occur when taking certain medicines.

For instance, while the predictable and beneficial effect of a narcotic is to relieve pain, one of its side effects is sleepiness. You are often informed of the side effects of common medications when they are prescribed.

As you are aware, chemotherapy works by damaging cells that are dividing frequently. But other noncancerous cell populations in the body are also dividing frequently. These are cells of the bone marrow (where blood cells are made) and the mucous membranes of the gastrointestinal (GI) tract (from the mouth to the large intestines). Hair follicles also divide quickly and are sensitive to some chemotherapy medicines. The side effects of chemotherapy reflect the effect that anticancer medicine has on all fast-growing cell populations. Most chemotherapy medicines temporarily affect the ability of the bone marrow to produce blood cells, including the white blood cells that fight infection. Some chemotherapy medicines temporarily cause gastrointestinal disturbances such as diarrhea or nausea and vomiting. Some chemotherapy medicines cause temporary hair loss or hair thinning.

The kind of side effects you may experience depends on the kind of chemotherapy drugs you are getting, the dose, and the frequency of your treatments. Your doctor and nurse will tell you what you can expect. It is most important to remember that chemotherapy's side effects (the disruption to healthy cells) are time limited and temporary. Some side effects are preventable. For instance, the side effect of nausea can often be prevented by taking antinausea medication before you start taking an anticancer drug and for several doses afterwards. Some side effects cannot be prevented, but there are many things that you can do to minimize, relieve, or manage them. Preventing and managing the side effects of chemotherapy is a very important part of your treatment plan and will help you live a normal, active life. Your GI system, hair, and blood cell–producing capabilities will return to normal after your treatments are over.

Chapters 5 through 10 will tell you much more about the possible side effects of chemotherapy and radiation therapy and how to cope with them. They explain why the side effects occur and how to prevent, relieve, or manage the problems if they develop.

2

What Is Radiation Therapy?
by Myles E. Lampenfeld, M.D.

In order to understand radiation therapy, you may find it helpful to understand what radiation is, where it comes from, and how it kills cancer cells. But first, a short lesson about atoms. This might be familiar if you ever studied chemistry in high school.

Atoms are the smallest chemical building blocks. They are made up of particles called protons, neutrons, and electrons. Protons and neutrons form a nucleus. Electrons orbit around the nucleus like planets around the sun. The positively charged nucleus attracts the negatively charged electrons like a magnet.

Everything that exists is made up of atoms—the stars and planets, soil and minerals, plants and animals. When atoms join with other atoms they usually form a stable molecule. For example, two hydrogen atoms join with an atom of oxygen to form a molecule of water. Atoms of such elements as oxygen, carbon, iron, calcium, and hydrogen can also join with other atoms to form molecules.

In the late 1800s scientists discovered that some atoms were unstable. Their outer electrons could escape the nucleus, giving off energy that could interact with other things in the environment. One form of this energy is radiant energy or *radiation*.

In 1895 Wilhelm Conrad Roentgen experimented with a flow of electrons through a vacuum tube. He noticed that the flow of electrons caused a chemical that was lying nearby to glow. The letter "X" stands for the unknown, so it was incorporated into the name "X ray" to describe this phenomenon. In later experiments he saw that radiation could pass through objects and leave an image on photographic plates. He was able to take X ray photographs of the interior of metal objects, and also took the first X ray of a human body—the bones of his wife's hand.

The first use of radiation for medical purposes started with an accident. In 1898 Marie and Pierre Curie discovered an element that gave off radiation naturally and called it radium. Henri Becquerel, another pioneer in the new field of radiation, was carrying a piece of radium in his vest pocket, and it caused a severe burn on his chest. It was this burn that led to exploration of how this radiant energy interacts with human cells, and how it could help treat diseases. Soon scientists were using both X rays and radium to treat skin cancer. The first report of a patient being cured by radiation was presented in 1899.

Types of Radiation

X rays, ultraviolet rays, and visible light are all part of the electromagnetic spectrum; individual particles of these are called *photons*. They are all forms of energy that travel in waves at the speed of light. Different kinds of electromagnetic rays have different characteristic wave frequencies (how frequently waves repeat their patterns) and wavelengths (how long the waves are). The shorter the waves, the more frequently they repeat, and the more energy they have. X rays, for example, have shorter wavelengths, higher frequency, and more energy than visible light.

Low-Energy X Rays

When you have a diagnostic X ray (like routine chest or dental X rays), a small burst of low-energy radiation harmlessly passes through your body. You cannot see or feel it, and this burst leaves an image on film. The image shows not only your shape but also shadows of your internal structures. The radiologist knows how normal bones, lungs, or intestines appear on an X-ray film and can sometimes identify problems or diseases if the shadows appear abnormal. A broken bone, a distortion in the shape of the stomach, or an abnormal collection of fluid in the lungs shown on X-ray films are all apparent to the radiologist who is an expert in interpreting the X ray images.

High-Energy X Rays

High-energy X rays can be used for radiation therapy because they are capable of penetrating the surface of your body. Although all energy waves (or parts of the electromagnetic spectrum) are useful, only X rays have sufficient energy to be used in cancer treatments. While low-energy X rays (like routine chest X rays or dental films) can harmlessly pass through the body, creating a photographic image, the high-energy X rays directed to the tumor damage the cells they come in contact with.

When high-energy radiation enters the body, it interacts with the atoms and molecules in the cell. The radiation, when directed to tumor cells, damages vital structures such as the tumor cell's DNA or enzymes. Some tumor cells die immediately, and some are so damaged that they can not divide (reproduce) and will die later. Cells are generally more vulnerable to the lethal effects of radiation when they are dividing. Because cancer cells divide more frequently than normal cells, they are more likely to be damaged by radiation than are normal cells.

How Radiation Is Produced

Most modern radiation therapy departments today use a high-energy form of X rays produced by a special machine called a *linear accelerator*. This machine accelerates electrons, which then bounce off a metal target and produce X rays. Faster electrons have higher energy and produce higher-energy X rays.

Linear accelerators also produce electron beams for radiation therapy. (Electrons are not photons and cannot penetrate the body as deeply as X rays can.) The electron beam is produced by removing the metal target from the path of the accelerated electrons. This kind of radiation therapy is often used for skin cancer. Electron beam "boosts" are sometimes useful for delivering additional radiation to the "tumor bed" (the area where the tumor was growing) following a course of penetrating photon radiation.

Radiation therapy can also use other parts of the atom. "Heavy particle" radiation uses the neutrons or protons (which are found in the center of the atom) and are much larger than electrons. These heavy particles are produced by a machine called a cyclotron. "Proton beam" therapy uses a more precise beam than an X ray beam. "Neutron beam" therapy uses a beam with different characteristics than X rays and may have advantages for tumors resistant to standard X rays. Neutrons have been used to treat prostate and salivary gland tumors.

There are other kinds of photons that are also used in radiation therapy. Gamma rays behave like X rays but are produced by radioactive elements such as radium and cesium.

Dividing the Dose—Fractionation

The goal of radiation treatment is to deliver the radiation beam at a dose that will prevent tumor cells from growing, but will allow normal cells to recover. The total dose of radiation will not be given all at once. A fraction of the total dose will be given with each treatment. This is called *fractionation*. A course of treatment usually requires two to eight weeks (with treatments five days a week). This adds up to ten to forty treatments over that period of time.

Fractionation has a number of advantages. First, a small dose of radiation given each day allows the normal cells in the surrounding area to recover. Second, since cells are more sensitive to the damaging effects of radiation when they are dividing, small daily treatments provide more opportunities to catch the frequently dividing cancer cells at that vulnerable time. Third, cancer cells are more vulnerable to the damaging effects of radiation when they have a good supply of oxygen carried by the blood. As the tumor shrinks over the weeks of treatment, the remaining tumor cells can get more blood, more oxygen, and thus become more sensitive to the effects of radiation.

Radiation Delivery

When the source of radiation is outside your body, it is called *external beam irradiation*. You are not radioactive. The radiation passes through you. It does not stay in the tumor, your blood, or any of your secretions.

The radiation oncologist, who specializes in the use of radiation to treat cancer, plans your treatment carefully. He or she uses diagnostic scans and computers to plan the beam arrangement to deliver most of the radiation to the tumor and avoid normal cells in the vicinity. This allows very precise placement of the beams.

When the source of the radiation is placed within your body, it is called *brachytherapy*. This kind of radiation treatment uses placement of the radiation source close to the tumor. Radioactive elements such as cesium, iridium, iodine, gold, phosphorus, and palladium have been used for brachytherapy.

When this type of therapy was first developed, the radioactive sources were put in the form of pellets, wires, or ribbons. A specific applicator was used to fit to the part of the body being treated, and then the radioactive source was inserted by the radiation oncologist. Treatment usually required two or more days, during which the patient was said to be "loaded," or radioactive, since the radioactive source was temporarily inside the body. The patient had to remain in the hospital isolated from other patients. This treatment was called low-dose brachytherapy.

In the last fifteen years high-dose (rate) brachytherapy (HDR) has largely replaced low-dose (rate) brachytherapy. HDR uses a highly active source, such as iridium, that gives off a large amount of radiation over a short time. This treatment may only take ten minutes instead of several days. The iridium source is programmed by a computer to be placed in the body then withdrawn automatically. This can be done as an outpatient in the radiation therapy department. Like other kinds of radiation, the total dose is divided so that a fraction is given each day. That allows time for normal tissue to recover between treatments. HDR is widely used for treatment of cancers of the cervix, endometrium, prostate, lung, esophagus, head, and neck.

Starting Treatment

If your oncologist believes that radiation therapy will be helpful, you will be referred to a radiation oncologist. The doctor will examine you and review your records, reports, and all relevant information. He or she will consider your general health, any other illnesses or treatments you may have had in the past, and the type and stage of the cancer. Additional tests may be needed.

The treatment plan will be based on the radiation oncologist's vast knowledge of the uses and effects of radiation and his or her prior experience treating similar patients with similar cancers, as well as new information reported in scientific journals and professional conferences. Treatment choices are always changing as new information and technology develop. Clinical trials test and compare different treatments and establish new standards. For instance, the standard treatment for breast cancer used to be a mastectomy (surgical removal of the breast). Clinical trials showed that for some women with breast cancer, lumpectomy (removal of the tumor only) along with radiation therapy is as effective a treatment option as a mastectomy.

When you meet with the radiation oncologist you will discuss the recommended treatment plan. Radiation therapy, like all treatments, has inherent risks and benefits. You need to know what they are. Your radiation oncologist will discuss the answers to these questions with you:

- What are the goals of treatment?
- How long will the treatment last?
- What can you expect in terms of relief of symptoms?
- What can you expect in terms of the possibility of improvement, remission, or cure?
- What are the short-term and long-term side effects of treatment?
- What are the possible complications?

Your medical oncologist, radiation oncologist, and primary care physician work together to monitor you while you are getting the therapy. They will continue to check your blood tests, diagnostic scans, and X rays to make sure that the treatment is working as expected.

The Planning Phase—Simulation

Next the radiation oncologist determines the exact area that needs radiation treatment, your body's position during the treatment, the dose of radiation, and how you will receive it. This preparation is called *simulation*. You will not receive radiation treatment during simulation, but everything will be prepared so that treatment can begin at another visit. Your simulation appointment could be as short as a half hour, or it may take several hours depending on the complexity of the plan. Simulation consists of five steps:

1. **Determining the Treatment Field**

   The *treatment field* is the area of your body that will receive radiation. It may include the tumor area alone, or it may also include lymph nodes found near that area. For instance, the treatment field for breast cancer usually consists of the entire breast. It may also include the lymph nodes under the arm and above the collarbone on the same side of the body. The treatment field for prostate cancer includes the entire prostate gland and may also include lymph nodes in the pelvis. Sometimes the treatment field may change during the course of treatment in order to protect a sensitive area or to deliver a higher dose to an area where it is needed.

2. **Determining the Technique**

   The radiation oncologist selects the kind of radiation beam to be used and how the radiation will be directed to the tumor or treatment field. This is called the *technique*. A skin cancer may need only one beam of radiation. Prostate cancer may be treated by six beams directed at the prostate from six different directions. The goal is to deliver a uniform dose of radiation to the tumor.

3. **Marking the Skin**

   The treatment field is then marked on the skin and recorded with X rays. The skin markings are lines drawn with ink. Near the end of the simulation session, the ink marks on your skin may be replaced with permanent tattoos. Tattoos are helpful because they precisely mark the treatment field, and they can't be washed off. They are made by putting a drop of ink on your skin and pricking the skin with a small needle, allowing a tiny spot of ink to flow into your skin. The excess ink is wiped off, and the tiny black dot remains.

4. **Shaping the Field—Blocking**

   Beams produced by radiation equipment are rectangular. Modern radiation equipment can produce a beam as small as 5x5 cm (2x2 in) or as large as 40x40 cm (15x15 in). The length and width of the beam will vary as needed. For instance, a beam aimed at the spine may be long and narrow while a beam used for treating an eye will be small and nearly square.

During the planning phase, the beam must be shaped to the exact dimensions of the area that needs treatment and exclude any area that does not require treatment. That is done by creating blocks that are made of an alloy. One such alloy is called *cerrobend*, which can be melted and poured into a Styrofoam mold of any shape. The radiation oncologist draws the shape of the blocks onto an X ray film of the treatment area, and then the mold is made. When the blocks are attached to the machine producing the radiation beam, the result is an irregular beam (instead of a rectangular beam) that conforms exactly to the treatment field.

Blocks are also used to protect some areas of your body which may be particularly sensitive to the effects of radiation. For instance, the spinal cord may need to be blocked after it has received a specific dose of radiation but before the treatments are completed. Eyes, the optic nerve, the heart, and kidneys are other critical structures that sometimes are blocked or excluded from part or all of a treatment course. If blocks are added or changed partway through the treatments, the simulation process may need to be repeated.

5. Positioning

The radiation oncologist uses different devices to ensure that your position does not shift during treatment, and that your body is in the same exact position each day. Plaster casts, sand bags, and other devices are used to support parts of your body, and make your position more precise and more comfortable during treatment. When the head, brain, face, or neck are radiated, sometimes a fitted face mask is created to comfortably hold your head in position during treatment.

When all the measuring, blocking, positioning, and calculating are complete, X rays of the treatment field are taken to assure that the daily treatment is exactly as the radiation oncologist planned. This is called *simulation verification* and usually takes place on the third visit to the radiation department.

Side Effects of Radiation Therapy

Unlike chemotherapy, which travels through your blood system to every cell in your body, the therapeutic effects and the side effects of radiation therapy are limited to the part of your body that is receiving treatment. Before any treatment begins, it is important to know what side effects to expect. You also need to know why they are happening, when they are likely to occur, and what you can do to prevent, minimize, or relieve the side effects.

The side effects associated with radiation are usually temporary, develop gradually over the weeks of your treatment, and resolve gradually after treatment has been completed. In general, more severe side effects are associated with larger doses of radiation, longer treatments, and a larger treatment field. Side effects may be more severe if you are getting chemotherapy and radiation therapy at the same time.

Prevention and relief of potential side effects is a very important part of your treatment. If you can feel good, stay well nourished, and continue your normal activities as much as possible, you will be able to complete therapy. The physician and nurses in the radiation department will be checking with you frequently to see how they can help you get through this treatment period. If problems develop, don't try to treat them yourself. Let your doctor or nurse know immediately so they can help prevent complications and relieve the symptoms as soon as possible.

Fatigue

Fatigue is the most common side effect of radiation therapy. Fatigue probably occurs because your body is working hard to eliminate tumor cells killed by the treatment and repair damage to normal cells. Like many other side effects of radiation treatments, you may not notice it immediately, but it develops gradually during the weeks of your therapy. After the treatments are completed, it will take several weeks for the fatigue to gradually lift and your energy to return.

Rest is essential, as well as maintaining good nutrition. During this time you may need even more calories and protein than usual in your diet. This is not the time to go on a weight reduction diet! Chapter 9 ("Coping with Fatigue") has more information about the fatigue associated with cancer treatments along with some suggestions about how to pace yourself while you are experiencing this symptom.

Skin Reactions—Dermatitis

All radiation passes through the skin surface on the way to treating the tumor. So it is no surprise that skin inflammation, or *dermatitis*, is a very common side effect of radiation therapy. In some ways it is similar to sunburn. Radiation can cause the skin to be itchy, dry, flushed, warm, or uncomfortable. The skin exposed to the radiation may get darker than your normal color. Dermatitis can also develop in the skin on the opposite side of the treatment field. This is because some of the radiation goes through the body and exits on the other side. This is called *exit dermatitis*. Exit dermatitis is more common when the radiation beam passes through a thin part of your body, such as the neck, and less common when it passes through a thicker part of your body, such as the chest.

Preventing or Minimizing Dermatitis

Your radiation oncologist will plan your treatment using skin-sparing techniques to prevent skin damage as much as possible. These techniques use higher energy X rays, which go some distance into and through the skin before depositing their maximum dose. The angle of the radiation beam also affects the severity of the skin reaction.

Another way to minimize skin irritation is to approach the tumor from several directions. This is called a *multifield technique*. This technique uses different radiation beams coming from different angles, all focused on the tumor. It helps prevent dermatitis because any one skin area receives only part of the total radiation dose that is directed at the tumor.

The most important thing you can do to prevent damage and protect the delicate skin in the treatment area is to avoid anything irritating. Sun exposure can do real damage to the skin and should be avoided as much as possible. The radiated skin area should always be covered with soft clothing if possible, or with sun block of at least SPF 15. A hat with a wide brim can protect your head, face, neck, or upper chest—areas that are not easily covered with clothing.

Avoid skin products that contain alcohol, as they can cause excessive drying to skin already dry from the radiation. Some fragrances (perfume, aftershave lotion, etc.) contain alcohol and are irritating. Chlorinated water in swimming pools, hot tubs, or spas may worsen radiation dermatitis. Bath or shower water that is too hot can also be irritating.

Healing Skin Problems

Your radiation oncologist or nurse may recommend skin products that are soothing and promote healing. Aloe vera is popular and effective, as are many moisturizing ointments, gels, creams, and lotions. Cornstarch is also soothing because it helps keep skin dry in the skin fold (under breasts, under arms, or in groin areas). If your skin reaction is severe, the radiation oncologist may recommend medications such as topical steroids (hydrocortisone), or topical antibiotics (Neosporin or Silvadene). Your radiation treatment may need to be delayed for a few days to allow your skin to heal.

Do not try to manage your skin reaction without professional input. Let the radiation oncologist or nurse assess the problem early and recommend the best products to protect or heal your skin.

Mouth Soreness—Mucositis

Mucositis is the irritation of the mucous membranes that line the mouth, throat, esophagus, and the rest of the digestive tract. The mucous membrane cells are very sensitive to the effects of radiation because they divide frequently. If the treatment field includes the mouth or neck you may develop inflammation and soreness of these membranes. Your mouth could feel sore or dry, or it may become painful to swallow, making it difficult to eat and drink normally. Inflammation of the mucous membranes can also make them more susceptible to a yeast infection (thrush) or a herpes infection (cold sores).

Chemotherapy can also cause mucositis. If you are getting both radiation and chemotherapy at the same time, it could make the problem of mucositis more severe. Mucositis, like the other side effects of radiation, may develop gradually over the course of your treatment, and it will clear up gradually after your treatment is completed.

Dealing with Mucositis

During the period of time when your mucous membranes are vulnerable to inflammation and infection, your should avoid anything that may irritate them further. Avoid alcohol and cigarettes, as well as very hot and very cold food and drinks. Rough or abrasive food such as crusty bread or toast may also be painful to the delicate tissues and should be avoided. Eat cool or warm food of soft or smooth textures (yogurt, mashed potatoes), which are tolerated better. See Chapter 6 ("Coping with Other Digestion Problems") and Chapter 7 ("Maintaining Good Nutrition") for more suggestions about mouth care and nutrition during this time.

Keeping your teeth and gums clean can really help prevent secondary infections and promote speedy healing of the mucous membranes. It is important to brush and floss after each meal and before bed time because food particles collecting on the teeth harbor bacteria. During the time when your gums are sore, use a soft toothbrush, brush carefully, and be very gentle when you floss. Rinse with a warm baking soda solution (1/2 tsp. of baking soda in 1/2 cup of warm water) to neutralizes the acid secretions in your mouth.

If pain is a problem, the doctor may order an anesthetic mouth rinse (like Xylocaine) to numb the inside of your mouth and throat. Antacids are soothing and counteract the effect of stomach acid on the esophagus. Antihistamines such as Benadryl are sometimes prescribed to prevent inflammation. Fungal and yeast infections of the mouth are treated with an antifungal liquid (such as nystatin), which you rinse with four to five times a day to coat the mucous membranes and relieve the problem. If you have a herpes infection in the mouth (cold sores) you may be given an antiviral medication (like acyclovir).

Look inside your mouth. Watch for sore spots, white patches, or blisters on your gums and inside your cheeks and lips. It's important to treat the problem of mucositis early. Let the physician or nurse know if your mouth and throat are becoming sensitive or painful, or if you are having trouble eating and drinking adequately. They can see if you are developing any infections and can start treatment to relieve the symptoms immediately.

Diarrhea

The small intestines are lined with cells that are dividing frequently. Therefore they are particularly sensitive to radiation. Since the small intestines fill the lower part of your abdomen, any radiation to the lower abdomen or pelvis could result in inflammation of the lining. When those cells become inflamed they produce more water and mucus than they normally do, which results in a change in the normal pattern of your bowel movements. Mild inflammation could cause your stools to be more frequent or very soft, and more severe inflammation could cause frequent watery stools, along with abdominal cramping, gas, and bloating.

The lining of the small intestines is designed to absorb fluids, nutrients, and essential electrolytes that your body needs to function. Diarrhea can cause these electrolytes (potassium, chloride, and sodium) to be lost along with too much water and mucus. Frequent large, watery stools can lead to dehydration, malnutrition, and an imbalance of these electrolytes. Eating can sometimes stimulate more diarrhea, but cutting down on your food and fluid can lead to even more dehydration. You need fluids, calories, and protein so your body can recover from the radiation treatments.

Prevention and Treatment of Diarrhea

If you are receiving radiation therapy that is likely to cause diarrhea, the radiation oncologist will probably recommend a bulk-forming fiber right from the start. Metamucil is a natural, partially-indigestible vegetable fiber that promotes regular bowel movements by absorbing the water in the small intestines. It also gives the stool more bulk, promotes more complete emptying, and doesn't allow irritating substances normally present in stool (such as bile acids) to dwell.

Diet modification such as a bland, low-fiber diet can help. Avoid caffeine, alcohol, and raw or greasy foods, which can stimulate more diarrhea. Some people find that eliminating dairy products temporarily is useful in controlling diarrhea. Foods that are high in carbohydrates such as potatoes, rice, or pasta are easily digested and are less likely to stimulate the intestines. See Chapter 7 ("Maintaining Good Nutrition") for more suggestions on how to eat and what foods to avoid if you have diarrhea.

If diarrhea continues to be a problem, your radiation oncologist may recommend antidiarrhea medication such as Lomotil or Imodium to slow down movement of the digestive tract. Even though these medicines are now available without a prescription, you should always check with the physician before taking them. Diarrhea could also be a sign that you have an infection in the bowel. The diarrhea could be the result of your intestines attempting to eliminate the toxins produced by the infecting organism.

Your doctor may want to send a sample of the diarrhea stool to the lab to identify the organism, then order a medication to eradicate the infection.

If diarrhea is severe and cannot be controlled with dietary measures and medicines, your radiation treatments may have to be delayed for a few days to give your intestines time to recover. You may also need IV fluids and electrolytes if the diarrhea is severe and prolonged. Like the other side effects of radiation therapy, diarrhea will slowly resolve a few weeks after radiation treatments are completed.

Nausea

Not everyone who has radiation therapy experiences nausea. It is usually only a problem if the stomach is within the treatment field. The stomach is most likely to be affected by abdominal radiation. It also can be affected by the exit radiation of a nearby area such as the spine (radiation could pass through the stomach on its way out of the body.)

Brain radiation can also cause nausea. There are structures deep within the brain that can cause nausea and vomiting when stimulated. This area may be stimulated by various events such as certain sights or smells, the feeling of stomach fullness, or the chemicals released by the body in response to some chemotherapy drugs. Radiation can also stimulate this area and cause nausea.

Some people are more affected by nausea associated with radiation therapy than others, just as there are some people more likely to develop seasickness, motion sickness, or morning sickness than others. Some people experience nausea without vomiting. If you have had recent surgery or chemotherapy you may be more predisposed to developing nausea from radiation therapy. In general, the larger the abdominal area being radiated, and the larger the dose of radiation, the more likely you would be affected by this side effect.

Prevention and Relief of Nausea

Prevention and relief of nausea is a very important part of your treatment. Nausea with or without vomiting is tremendously debilitating. When you are feeling nauseated, you can hardly think or do anything else. If you are nauseated, you cannot eat and drink or even rest adequately. Prevention is the key. Fortunately there are many effective medications now available to prevent most nausea, or to relieve it if it occurs.

Medications. If it is likely that you will experience nausea associated with your radiation treatments, the radiation oncologist will prescribe antinausea medications to take even before your treatment begins. Compazine or Tigan are usually prescribed first. You will be instructed to take the medication before your radiation treatment, and at set intervals as needed during the day. If those medications are not effective or not tolerated, there are other medications available. Zofran or Kytril are newer antinausea medicines that are now available in a pill form, and are very helpful in relieving nausea and vomiting. Reglan is sometimes recommended to speed up the digestive system to help the stomach empty faster. Reglan will not be prescribed if you are also having diarrhea, because in that case the digestive system may already be moving things out too quickly.

Dietary Measures. A bland diet is generally easier to digest when you are trying to minimize nausea. Avoid strong flavors or strong aromas that will stay with you and trigger nausea. Avoid fatty or spicy foods, coffee, or alcohol. Small, frequent meals are better tolerated than great heaps of food. Some people experience very mild nausea and find that snacking frequently during the day helps relieve it without medication. Chapter 5 ("Coping with Nausea") explains the problem of nausea as well as giving you many suggestion about how to cope and feel better. Chapter 7 ("Maintaining Good Nutrition") has dietary suggestions that will be useful as well.

Be a Detective. Everybody is unique in how they react to radiation treatment and what works to give them relief. Pay attention to the pattern of your nausea, and what helps you feel better. Then create a strategy that works for you. The following questions will help you to analyze your pattern:

- Do you feel nauseated before, during, or immediately after treatment?

- Do you feel nauseated several hours after treatment?

- Do you feel more or less nauseated if you eat before treatment?

- Does it make the nausea worse if you feel hungry?

- Does it help to take the antinausea medication before the treatment?

- Does it help to try to sleep immediately after the treatment?
- What medications work best?
- What foods do you crave?
- Does mild physical activity such as taking a walk help relieve the problem?

Hair Loss

At the base of your hair shaft, in the hair follicle, there are rapidly dividing cells that make your hair grow. Radiation therapy damages those cells and causes hair loss in those areas exposed to radiation. Hair loss can also occur on the opposite side of the body because of exit radiation. For instance, radiation treatment of one side of the head may cause hair loss on both sides because some of the radiation will go all the way through and affect the hair follicles on the opposite side. You will notice hair loss after a few weeks of treatment

Depending on the dose of radiation, hair loss may be temporary or permanent. Your radiation oncologist will tell you whether or not you can expect your hair to regrow, and when that will start to happen. Even if you know that your hair loss is temporary, you still have to deal with the problem until it grows back. Many people are able to camouflage patches of baldness on their head by growing hair in the adjacent areas a little longer.

The hair on your head keeps your head warm and protects your scalp from the sun. If there are large areas of hair loss on the head, even temporarily, you need to be sure to protect those areas from sun exposure or extreme cold. Use sunblock, a hat, or scarf when out in the elements. See Chapter 8 ("Coping with Hair Loss and Skin Changes") for more information.

Inflammation of the Bladder—Cystitis

Radiation therapy to the bladder can cause the cells lining the bladder to become inflamed. This inflamation is called *cystitis.* As with other side effects of radiation, the larger the treatment field and the larger the dose of radiation, the more likely this problem will develop. Radiation of the organs in the pelvis, such as the treatment of prostate cancer or cancer of the endometrium (lining of the uterus), can cause cystitis.

When the bladder lining becomes inflamed, you may have the urge to urinate frequently. Your bladder may feel full with only a small amount of urine inside. You may feel burning during urination, or see a small amount of blood in the urine. Fortunately cystitis does not usually cause a loss of urinary control.

Relieving the Symptoms

Although cystitis is a temporary problem that will gradually improve after your radiation treatments are completed, there are things you can do to feel better. For instance, you can increase the amount of fluid in your diet, since urine that is very concentrated is more irritating when the lining of the bladder is inflamed. Your radiation oncologist may prescribe Pyridium, a medicine that acts as bladder anesthetic. Pyridium decreases the bladder inflammation and relieves the urge to urinate frequently.

Complications of Radiation Therapy

Complications of radiation therapy occur when healthy cells are damaged by their exposure to the radiation. It would be ideal if radiation could be directed to tumor area alone and no other structures or organs would be affected at all. Although your radiation oncologist tries to plan your treatment so there is a minimum exposure of healthy cells to the radiation, completely protecting these cells is not yet possible. Before treatment begins, your radiation oncologist will tell you of the possible short-term and long-term complications of radiation treatments.

When complications do occur they are usually specific to the treated area. For instance, approximately 2 percent of the people who have had pelvic or abdominal irradiation develop complications that can cause bowel obstruction. During the course of treatment the small bowel may become inflamed from the radiation and then become scarred, leading to a loss of normal flexibility. An obstruction or blockage of the small bowel may then occur months or years later and may require surgery to correct. Breast irradiation occasionally results in a form of lung damage that can lead to a chronic cough or shortness of breath. This can occur because a small area of lung was exposed to the radiation during treatment. The risk is small but present.

As mentioned before, the larger the radiation field, and the larger the dose of radiation received, the greater the chance of having a complication develop later on. Preexisting illnesses such as diabetes, heart disease, or previous abdominal surgeries can increase the risk of developing complications.

Your radiation oncologist does many things to minimize the risk of developing complications. Careful blocking and treatment planning help make treatment safer. Giving a fraction of the radiation dose each day (fractionation) over a long period of time also reduces the risk. The radiation oncologist has to find a balance between the amount of radiation that is effective in eradicating disease and the risk of causing damage to healthy tissues.

Radiation therapy plays a very important role in cancer treatment. Although it is a highly technical and seemingly mysterious medical specialty, radiation therapy has been an effective treatment for some kinds of cancer for many years. As the technology develops it will become an even more precise and effective treatment in the future. Understanding how the therapy works, what to expect, and how to manage side effects caused by the treatment will help you be better prepared to cope with the problems that arise and to get help when you need it.

About the Author

Myles Lampenfeld, M.D., was born in Pennsylvania, where he began his training. He was board-certified in internal medicine and medical oncology before earning board-certification in radiation oncology. He began practice as a radiation oncologist twelve years ago in Berkeley, California. Dr. Lampenfeld is interested in the treatment of benign as well as malignant disease with radiation. He finds direct patient care gratifying and enjoys the technical aspects of his specialty.

3

Understanding
Blood Tests

When you are ill, it seems that everyone is after your blood. Every time you look up there's someone in a lab coat, carrying a tourniquet and multicolored test tubes, who needs just a few more ounces. You probably wonder "Why so many tests? Why so often?" You may even feel that you are giving too much blood and worry how and when your body will replace it.

You have about four to five quarts of blood in your body, and most blood tests require only about a teaspoon of blood in each test tube. The few teaspoons of blood you lose each time blood is drawn for a test are rapidly replaced. Even someone donating a pint of blood replaces it so quickly that he or she can donate again in about two weeks.

This chapter covers some of the most frequent blood tests that your doctor may order. Many of them can be done at the same time, with only one needle stick. The nurse or lab technicians can simply keep the needle in place and change the collection tubes. Then the samples can be sent to different departments in the lab for analysis. Unfortunately, there are times (especially when you are a patient in the hospital) when, as soon as the lab technician leaves, another comes in for another test and another needle stick. But as a rule, your doctors and nurses try to consolidate the tests so that doesn't happen.

In the hospital, routine blood tests are usually drawn very early in the morning, around five o'clock. This is a source of great annoyance to many people, since they can't imagine why samples must be taken at such an ungodly hour. The reason blood samples are collected so early is that it takes several hours for the lab to perform all the tests and get the results to the nurse's station and into your chart. When the doctors come each day to review your chart and determine what medications, IVs, treatments, or tests you need, the results of blood tests are an important source of information.

Don't hesitate to ask your nurse or doctor what blood tests are being done and why they are necessary. You also may want to know the results of the tests and what they indicate about your condition. Some people even keep notes about their blood tests—which tests were done, why they were done, and the results.

Why Test Your Blood?

Blood is the fluid of life. It carries oxygen from your lungs to each and every cell of your body. It carries the glucose that all your cells need for energy and then carries off the waste products from the cells' activities. Blood contains your body's defense against infection and carries the means of repairing the vessels (arteries and veins) in which it flows. Blood maintains the balance of all the chemicals that are necessary for muscles and nerves to function and provides the communication and coordination for all your organs to work together. With these diverse functions, you can see why a small sample of your blood provides an amazing window into the health and functioning of every organ. A mere teaspoon or two, when analyzed by the lab, can tell a great deal about you.

Blood is made of cells and plasma. The blood cells are red cells, white cells, and platelets, which are all produced in your bone marrow. The plasma is a straw-colored fluid containing blood cells along with glucose, electrolytes, enzymes, minerals, vitamins, hormones, and everything else your body needs to stay alive. A complete blood count (CBC) identifies the types, quantities, and characteristics of the different cells of your blood. A blood chemistry analyzes the plasma.

Bone Marrow—The Blood Cell Factory

Bone marrow is the tissue within your bones where blood cells are made. In infants, all the bone marrow is capable of manufacturing blood cells. But in adults, blood cells are made only in the flat bones such as the pelvis, sternum (breast bone), vertebrae, and skull.

The bone marrow is like a blood cell factory. It contains stem cells that have the capacity to evolve into all three types of blood cells. A stem cell can develop into a red blood cell and carry oxygen. Or it can evolve into a white blood cell and fight infection. Or it can evolve into a platelet, which can stop bleeding by forming a clot.

Bone marrow maintains the normal number of the three types of cells by replacing old cells as they naturally die off and increasing production of any kind of blood cell if there is a special demand for it. For instance, your bone marrow will step up production of white blood cells when you have an infection.

The bone marrow is a place where cells are dividing very quickly in order to keep up with your body's constant demand for blood cells of all kinds. Since chemotherapy and radiation therapy affect the cells that are dividing quickly (like cancer cells), it will temporarily affect your bone marrow. Unlike cancer cells, your bone marrow will recover and resume its normal production of blood cells.

Chemotherapy and radiation therapy do not affect the blood cells that are already in circulation, since they are not dividing. Only the production of new cells in the bone marrow is slowed down. Chemotherapy's effect on your bone marrow usually shows up in your blood cell count about a week to ten days after your treatment. That is when you can see that the blood cells have not been replaced at the normal rate. But in another week or so, the number of blood cells in circulation will return to normal.

Your chemotherapy treatments are timed to allow your bone marrow to recover. Your doctor will always check your blood cell count before each treatment to be sure that your bone marrow is back on the job of producing blood cells.

Radiation therapy will affect blood cell production only if the flat bones that are producing blood cells are exposed to the radiation. Even if the treatments are likely to cause a delay in the blood cell's production of your bone marrow, it will not be apparent for several weeks, since side effects of radiation therapy tend to be cumulative over time. Your radiation oncologist will check your blood counts periodically to keep track of how the treatments are affecting your bone marrow.

Red Blood Cells

Your red blood cells (also called *erythrocytes*) give your blood its color. Ninety percent of each red cell is made up of *hemoglobin*, a substance rich in iron. The size, shape, and flexibility of red cells enable them to squeeze through the small openings between cells. The red blood cells' purpose is to carry oxygen from your lungs to every corner of your body and carry carbon dioxide from the cells to your lungs to be exhaled. If you have too few red blood cells because of blood loss or because your bone marrow is not working normally, then your body's ability to carry oxygen and carbon dioxide is jeopardized. This condition is called *anemia.*

When your red blood cell count is low, your heart has to work harder to cycle the remaining red cells at a faster rate to provide your body with the oxygen it needs. You may feel tired, since there may not be enough oxygen to keep up with the activity of your muscles. You may feel dizzy when you stand up after you have been sitting or lying down. You may chill more easily or feel more winded after exerting yourself. These are all symptoms indicating that your body needs more oxygen and more red blood cells to carry it.

Red blood cells have a relatively long life span (about three or four months). While the production of new cells may be temporarily slowed down, the fact that they live so long makes the problem much less severe. By the time more cells are needed, your bone marrow has long since recovered and has usually caught up.

A complete blood count (CBC) provides three measurements that reflect the adequacy of your red blood cells. They are the red blood cell count (RBC), hemoglobin (Hgb), and hematocrit (Hct).

The *red blood cell count* is the number of red blood cells in a cubic millimeter of blood. The normal amount of red blood cells is about four amd a half to six million per cubic millimeter for men and four to five and a half million per cubic millimeter for women. The normal values for women are less than for men because women who are menstruating lose a small amount of blood each month with their periods.

The *hemoglobin* (Hgb) *test* measures the amount of this substance in a sample of blood. Hemoglobin is the part of a red blood cell that actually carries the oxygen, so an Hgb test gives a good indication of the cells' ability to carry oxygen from the lungs to all the parts of your body. Normal hemoglobin for men is from fourteen to eighteen grams per 100 milligrams of blood. For women it is slightly less (twelve to sixteen grams).

The *hematocrit* (Hct) measurement determines what percent of the sample of whole blood contains red blood cells. Normally, red blood cells comprise 42 to 54 percent for men and 38 to 46 percent for women.

If you have lost a lot of blood or your red blood cell production has been slowed down, then all three tests will be lower than normal. As your body turns up the production of red blood cells in the bone marrow or you receive a blood transfusion, all three values will rise.

What to Do When Your Red Cell Blood Count Is Low

Many people get through chemotherapy without having a noticeable drop in the production of their red blood cells. Since the cells live for so long and the bone marrow recovers in four to ten days after chemotherapy, they are soon replaced. Depending on your general health, you may be able to cope with a mild drop in red blood cells without noticing anything more than fatigue. The following measures may be helpful:

- Eat a well-balanced diet, especially foods high in iron. Drink lots of fluids as well.

- Your doctor may prescribe an iron supplement.

- Take your time when getting up from a lying or sitting position. If you're dizzy, take some deep breaths until it subsides.

• Get plenty of rest. During this time it helps to pace your activities. If you have a lot to do, don't try get everything done at once. Take breaks to recover your energy before going on.

Stimulating Red Blood Cell Production

A special hormone stimulates bone marrow to produce red blood cells. This hormone, *erythropoietin*, is normally produced by the kidneys in response to a drop in the oxygen-carrying capacity of the blood. Erythropoietin works by stimulating the red blood cells to mature faster. A synthetic version of this hormone can be given by injection to speed up red blood cell production when it has been slowed by the effects of chemotherapy or radiation therapy. If you have a severe drop in your red blood cells, you may require a blood transfusion.

White Blood Cells

White blood cells (*leukocytes*) provide your body's defense from infection. They are produced and stored in the bone marrow and are released when the body needs them. Once in the bloodstream, they circulate for only about twelve hours. Any inflammation or bacterial invasion will attract these cells, triggering them to leave the bloodstream and gather at the site of infection. There they surround the bacteria or other foreign body, stretching and wrapping themselves around it and then digesting it. White blood cells also help damaged tissue repair itself.

There are five kinds of white blood cells that are produced in the bone marrow. The first three (*neutrophils, eosinophils,* and *basophils*) have a granular appearance when seen under a microscope, and because of this they are called *granulocytes*. The two other types are *lymphocytes* and *monocytes*.

Neutrophils. Neutrophils are the most numerous white blood cells. They comprise 62 percent of all white blood cells and are the first to gather at an infection. Their job is to localize and neutralize bacteria. Each neutrophil can inactivate from five to twenty bacteria. When neutrophils are used up from fighting bacteria, they rupture, and the contents of the ruptured cell attracts even more neutrophils, as well as increasing the blood supply to that area. The increased blood circulation can make an infected area appear redder and feel hotter than usual.

Eosinophils. Eosinophils are the white blood cells that respond to allergic reactions. Their job is to detoxify foreign proteins before they can harm the body. They also contain toxic granules that can kill invading cells and clean up areas of inflammation.

Basophils. Basophils, the rarest of the white blood cells, release *histamine*, which increases blood supply and attracts other white blood cells to the infected area. Basophils make it easier for white blood cells to migrate out of the blood into the damaged area. They also release *heparin*, which dissolves old clots.

Lymphocytes. Lymphocytes not only fight infection, but also provide you with immunity to certain diseases. For example, the measles virus has an *antigen*—a substance that your body recognizes as foreign. Lymphocytes react to that foreign substance by forming *antibodies*. Antibodies are proteins which are designed to kill one specific antigen. There are many kinds of antigens, and your lymphocytes develop many different kinds of antibodies to attack them. These antibodies not only fight the foreign substance, but remember it so they can kill it whenever you are exposed to it again. Even if it is many years after your first exposure, the antibodies made by your lymphocytes remember the antigen and provide immunity.

Lymphocytes can be produced by the bone marrow or by other organs, such as the lymph glands, spleen, tonsils, or the thymus gland. They move back and forth between your blood and your lymph system. While many lymphocytes produce antibodies, others function as regulators for your immune response, either helping it or suppressing it depending on how well you are fighting an infection.

Monocytes. The last type of white blood cells are the body's second line of defense because they do not respond as quickly as neutrophils. Their job is to move into an infected area to remove damaged or dying cells or cell debris. They contain special enzymes that are very effective in killing bacteria. Monocytes are produced in the bone marrow and initially circulate in your blood. Once they leave the blood, they go into the tissue and establish themselves in the lymph nodes, lungs, liver, or spleen.

Signs of Infection

All five kinds of white blood cells work together to fight infection. The usual signs of infection are swelling, redness, warmth in the affected area, and fever. These symptoms indicate that your immune system is working, fighting bacteria or other foreign organisms. The formation of pus in an infection is really a collection of old, dead bacteria and exhausted white blood cell debris.

Unlike red blood cells, which live for months, white blood cells have a life span of only three or four days, and the bone marrow is constantly producing new cells to replace them. It is the bone marrow's production of white blood cells that is most vulnerable to the effects of chemotherapy and radiation. The cells that are already in circulation or in your tissues are not affected because they are not dividing. But when these cells die off and the reserves have been used up (within one week after your chemotherapy, or after several weeks of radiation therapy), your white blood count reaches its lowest point. This period is called the *nadir*.

The nadir is the time when you are most susceptible to infection. If you are exposed to bacteria during that time, your immune system may not be able to make as strong a response because there are just fewer white blood cells to respond. Following the nadir, your bone marrow will begin to catch up with white blood cell production and your blood count will recover. Your white blood cell count returns to normal about three weeks after your chemotherapy, or several weeks after your radiation therapy treatments are over.

Your doctor expects your white blood cell count to drop temporarily, but he or she will always check it before continuing treatment. If there is a delay in recovery, your doctor may delay your treatment for a few days and then check your count again. After several chemotherapy treatments or several weeks of radiation therapy, it is not unusual for your white blood cell count to be a little sluggish in returning to normal.

What to Do When Your White Blood Cell Count Is Low

Many people who are getting chemotherapy weather the period when their white blood cell counts are low without problem. But you do need to take special precautions to avoid infection during this time. Here's what to do:

- Stay away from anyone who has a cold, flu, or other infection.

- Stay away from large crowds of people in an enclosed environment to avoid being exposed to coughs and sneezes.

- Keep your skin clean and dry. Moisture provides a breeding place for bacteria. You carry many germs on your hands, so be sure to wash your hands often, especially after using the toilet. Remind others (doctors, nurses, or anyone else helping with your care) to wash their hands too.

- Keep your teeth and gums clean, as the food left on your teeth or under your dentures is a place bacteria could grow.

- Drink plenty of fluids, since urinating frequently will keep your bladder from developing an infection.

- Take special care to wash and disinfect any break in your skin and let your doctor know about all cuts or burns. Since it is the action of your white blood cells that causes inflammation, redness, or pus, you may not have these familiar signs of infections while your white blood cell count is low. You may have an infection and not even know it!

- Check with your doctor if you have any signs of a cold, cough, flu, or fever during this time as well. He or she may want you to take an antibiotic to help your body fight infection more effectively.

When all your chemotherapy treatments are over, your body's defenses will return to normal. But during this time, any exposure or risk of infections should be treated aggressively.

Stimulating White Blood Cell Production

Special proteins in your body called *colony stimulating factor* (CSF) stimulate the production of white blood cells. New techniques in genetic engineering have produced different forms of this protein that can be given by injection to counteract the effects of cancer treatments on the body's immune system. The form of CSF that increases granulocytes is called G-CSF. When this stimulating factor is given, it causes your bone marrow to speed up the maturation and release of particular white blood cells and shortens the period of time that you are vulnerable to infection.

Not everyone getting chemotherapy will need this medicine to stimulate white blood cell production. But if there is a delay in bone marrow recovery or a high risk of infection, CSF can help your bone marrow recover sooner.

Infections

You are surrounded by a world you cannot see. All around you are bacteria, molds, yeast, and viruses that can only be observed under a microscope. Everything you touch or eat and even the lining of your digestive system is teeming with microorganisms that could cause infection if they were to penetrate into your blood or tissues.

It is your intact skin and mucous membranes that usually keep these microorganisms from invading your blood system. It is only when these natural barriers are compromised that you risk infection. Your immune system then becomes your next line of defense, mobilizing to fight the infection that has penetrated your skin or mucous membranes.

If an infection is severe or your immune system is compromised, you may need some help to fight it. Antibiotics are medicines that help your body fight bacterial infections. There are a number of different antibiotics, and some are more effective in killing certain bacteria than others. Your doctor may want to determine the exact bacteria that is causing your infection to prescribe the best antibiotic. He or she does this by ordering a culture.

Getting a Culture

You are probably familiar with throat cultures that determine what kind of organism is causing a sore throat. The doctor or nurse will take a sterile swab and wipe the back of your throat with it. Then the swab is smeared across a nutrient-rich gel and placed in a warm environment to encourage the bacteria to grow rapidly. In a day or two there are enough bacteria growing in the nutrient so that they can be examined under a microscope. The microbiologist in the lab can then see the exact bacteria causing the problem and determine which antibiotic will be most effective in killing it. When this test is done, it is called a *culture* (the process of growing the bacteria in a nutrient) and *sensitivity* (the process of determining which antibiotics are most effective in killing that bacteria). Viruses, molds, and yeast can be cultured as well.

Bacteria and other organisms can be cultured from anything your body produces, such as urine, sputum, stool, or drainage from wounds. Blood cultures are quite common. If you have a fever or any other sign of infection, your doctor may want to determine if bacteria (or other organisms) are present in your blood. A sample of your blood is taken and put in an environment which encourages microorganisms to grow. Since your blood supply is so large, it's often difficult to capture a particular organism in a small sample. Accordingly, you may have to have two samples of blood taken a few minutes apart to improve the chances of finding something.

If your infection is severe or your level of infection-fighting white blood cells is low, your doctor may not wait until the exact bacteria has been identified. After a sample of blood has been taken, he or she may want you to start taking an antibiotic right away. Usually your doctor will choose a broad spectrum antibiotic, named for its capacity to kill many different kinds of bacteria. In a few days, when the lab can identify the exact organism, your antibiotic may be changed to one that is more specific for that organism.

Fine-Tuning the Antibiotic

To fight infections successfully, you need the correct antibiotic at the correct dose for a long enough time to assure that the infection is gone. That is why your doctor and nurse will remind you to take all of the antibiotic prescribed, even though the signs and symptoms of infection seem to disappear after a day to two. Most antibiotic pills are prescribed for a week to ten days. More severe infections may require IV antibiotics for a few days, and then, depending on the organism and your response, you may be switched to pills, tablets, or capsules.

With some IV antibiotics, the dose must be fine-tuned to be sure it is effective against the infection, but not harmful to your body. The doctor, therefore, needs to know the antibiotic's *peak* and *trough*. The peak is the greatest amount of medicine in your system (right after you receive it), and the trough is the least amount in your system (right before the next dose). To determine the peak and trough, your blood will be drawn twice, both before and after you get the medication. With this information, your doctor can adjust the dose so you are getting the right amount.

Platelets

The cells in your blood that help to form a clot are called *platelets*. Platelets are produced in the bone marrow from a cell called a *megakaryocyte*.

Platelets help your body stop bleeding from nicks or cuts. They do that by collecting at the site of an injury and making the blood vessel constrict. Platelets then begin a series of chemical reactions that, along with other clotting factors in the liquid part of your blood, form a clot. After the vessel has healed and the clot has served its purpose, another series of chemical reactions causes the clot to dissolve so that the blood vessel is open again to carry blood.

Platelets are formed in large numbers, with as many as 150,000 to 300,000 in each cubic millimeter of blood. They live for about ten days in circulation. Chemotherapy slows down platelet production just as it slows down the production of all the other blood cells that are dividing frequently. The platelets in circulation are not affected because they aren't dividing, but formation of the megakaryocytes (which will become new platelets) may fall behind temporarily. The period of time when your platelet count is the lowest (the nadir) comes about ten to fourteen days after your chemotherapy or after several weeks of radiation therapy.

What to Do When Your Platelet Count Is Low

Many people get through all their chemotherapy treatments without being in danger of serious bleeding because of lack of platelets. Mostly it is a matter of being more careful to avoid injury and paying more attention to any bruise or abrasion.

During the nadir, you may find that you bruise more easily or bleed slightly longer from a cut or after a blood test. Here are a few things to watch for:

- Check your skin all over for bruising or broken blood vessels. Check with your doctor if a bruise continues to increase in size.

- Notify your doctor of nosebleeds or headaches.

- Avoid contact sports to prevent falls or injuries.

- Wear protective gloves when working in the yard.

- Use an electric razor instead of a blade to avoid cuts or nicks when shaving.

- Notify your doctor if you notice blood in your urine or stool.

- Brush and floss carefully since your mucous membranes are more likely to bleed during this time. Use a soft-bristle brush and a more gentle technique.

- Notify your doctor before any dental appointments.

- Notify your doctor before any appointments with other health care providers such as the chiropractor, acupuncturist, podiatrist, etc.

Plasma

Plasma is the fluid in which the red cells, white cells, and platelets circulate. It contains many substances that are essential for your body to function. For example, sodium, potassium, chloride, calcium, magnesium, and other elements must be present in your body in specific amounts. That's because salts from these elements, when dissolved, can carry an electric charge that enables your heart, nerves, and muscles to work properly. These elements are called *electrolytes*.

Electrolytes

Your kidneys help to regulate the balance of electrolytes by selectively eliminating or retaining these elements. For example, if you eat food that contains a high level of potassium, sodium, or calcium, your kidneys will keep what is needed and get rid of the excess. Chemotherapy treatments can temporarily affect your body's ability to keep a normal balance of electrolytes. Your doctor may therefore need to adjust the amount of electrolytes you get in your IV or take by mouth.

Proteins

There are also proteins in plasma. These are large molecules, such as *albumin* and *globulin*, whose presence controls the flow of fluid from the blood system to the cells. Low levels of albumin can occur with malnutrition. This may cause water and plasma to leak out of the veins into the surrounding tissue, causing swelling (edema).

Enzymes

Your heart and liver contain unique enzymes. If these organs have been damaged (from a heart attack or from liver damage), the enzyme specific to that organ can be detected at higher levels than normal in plasma. When the levels of these enzymes drop back to normal, it indicates that the organ is recovering.

Other Substances in Plasma

The levels of nitrogen, urea, and creatinine found in blood plasma indicate how well your kidneys are working. Since many chemotherapy drugs are excreted through your kidneys, your doctor will check the levels of these substances in your plasma to determine the drugs and the doses that are safe and effective for you.

There are also substances in plasma called *clotting factors*. They work with your platelets to form clots when needed and then work to dissolve the clots when they are no longer needed.

The amounts of glucose, protein, iron, and cholesterol in plasma can reflect your diet or digestion. An analysis of plasma can also provide early warning for diabetes, hormone imbalances, iron and vitamin deficiencies, or the risk of heart disease.

Testing plasma allows your doctor to check on how every organ is functioning. It is important to monitor not only how well the chemotherapy is working to kill cancer cells, but how the chemotherapy is affecting all the normal cells as well.

Tumor Markers

Research scientists are always looking for a simple blood test that will predict cancer at its earliest stage, as well as indicate how well the cancer treatments are working. This kind of test could also warn of recurrence long before there are any symptoms.

Although there is no current test that can accurately predict cancer's occurrence or cure, there are a number of substances in your blood whose presence at certain levels is associated with particular kinds of cancers. These substances are called *tumor markers*. Their levels tend to rise if the cancer is growing and drop when the cancer is destroyed.

If you have breast cancer, your doctor may be testing your blood for the tumor marker CA15-3 or CA27•29. The tumor marker CA-125 may be periodically checked if you have ovarian cancer.

An important drawback of tumor markers is that a rise in the tumor marker may not always be caused by cancer, but by another disease or condition. A rise in the prostatic-specific antigen (PSA) can indicate prostate infection as well as prostate cancer. A rise in the blood level of carcinoembryonic antigen (CEA) is associated with cancer of the colon, pancreas, breast, or intestines, but a rise in CEA may also occur with pancreatitis, inflammatory bowel disease, or emphysema. A rise in the enzyme prostatic acid phosphatase (PAP) is associated with cancer of the prostate, bone, or multiple myeloma. But a rise in PAP is also possible with osteoporosis.

In other words, tumor markers are not foolproof in their ability to predict the presence or absence of cancer. But they are one of many tools your doctor has in following your progress. Comparative X rays, scans, and physical examinations, along with changes in your tumor markers, are all ways the doctor can tell how your treatment is progressing.

Interfacing with Other Health Care Professionals

Let your doctor know if you are planning any other medical treatments. Visits to the dentist, podiatrist, or chiropractor should be cleared by your oncologist first. During the period of time when you have fewer white blood cells or platelets than normal, you are more likely to bruise or bleed easily, and you are less resistant to infections. Your oncologist will advise you when other treatments are safe and the kind of precautions that other doctors need to take during this time. For the same reason, let other health professionals know that you are receiving chemotherapy so that they will consider this when planning and scheduling their treatments.

Coping

Blood tests are so common and so useful in the diagnosis and treatment of diseases that medical people forget how stressful they may be for the patient. Here are some suggestions that may help you cope:

- It helps if you can relax. If you are not in a panic, your veins are easier to find. Make sure that you are comfortable and your arm is well supported. When your arm stays still, the needle causes less pain.

- If you can anticipate when the test will be done, you may want to ask for a warm blanket to wrap around your arms. The heat will make your veins swell and make it easier for the nurse or technician to take the blood sample.

- When the test is over, apply pressure to the vein for at least five minutes. This is especially important if your platelet count is low and your body takes longer to form a clot. Applying pressure will minimize the amount of bruising and pain you have afterwards.

4

The IV Experience

Nobody likes needles. No one likes to extend his or her arm and await the tourniquet and the cold swab of alcohol. You pray that your veins will stand out and fear that the worried look of the technician indicates that you and your veins might be a problem. People who are receiving chemotherapy have to face that moment of truth many times during their treatment. Frequent blood tests are important to monitor your response to cancer treatments, the recovery of your immune system, the functioning of your kidneys, the presence of infection, and so on. Besides the blood tests, most chemotherapy drugs are given intravenously (in the vein—IV for short). When medicine is sent into your vein, it's quickly distributed by the blood all through your body. Most chemotherapy drugs are not available in a form that you can swallow, because they may be damaging to the lining of your stomach or would be rendered less effective by the action of different gastrointestinal enzymes and secretions.

More about Veins

Veins and arteries are muscular tubes that respond by swelling or contracting in response to temperature, activity, or emotions. You can notice how prominent your veins get on a hot day or when you are playing baseball or kneading dough. You may have also noticed that your veins seem to disappear when you have been inactive, feel cold, or are anxious. Unfortunately, many people feel anxious when they are faced with needles while having an IV started or blood drawn. They find that their once prominent veins are nowhere to be seen. Closing down the blood circulation to arms and legs and shunting it to vital organs is a reflex that happens automatically when someone is afraid.

Fortunately, there are ways of getting veins to dilate and become more accessible. A tourniquet (the thick rubber band that is wrapped around your upper arm) partially constricts the veins and traps some blood in the arms and hands, which makes your veins stand out. Warming your arms or flexing your muscles by clenching and unclenching your fist are other ways that your veins will fill with blood and stand out.

Good Veins and Bad Veins

The ease or the difficulty that a nurse may have in starting your IV depends on a number of factors. The condition of your blood vessels (arteries and veins) reflects your general health and strength. Strong, young, muscular people tend to have strong, muscular blood vessels. Older people, as well as those who are ill or malnourished, have more fragile vessels. Frequent punctures and irritating medications such as antibiotics or chemotherapy can make veins temporarily less flexible and more tender and fragile. The skill and experience of the person approaching your veins is, of course, another factor. Starting an IV takes coordination, judgment, and skill. And the more experience that a person has, the fewer problems there will be with the procedure.

Which Vein?

Many different veins can be used to draw blood or start an IV if the veins are sufficiently large, close to the surface, and can be dilated by using a tourniquet. The tourniquet makes the veins easier to feel and see. After the blood sample has been collected or the IV started, the tourniquet is released and normal blood flow continues as before.

Blood samples are usually drawn from a large vein at the inside of your elbow. That vein, however, is rarely used in starting an IV because it would restrict the movement of your entire arm. In general, the veins in the back of your hand and the lower arm are best for IVs. They are visible and accessible, and the needle can be anchored (using tape) to prevent accidental removal without restricting your movement.

Needles

Short-Term IVs

The kind of needle used to start an IV depends on whether the IV will be used for a short time (just a few minutes) or over a longer period (several hours or days). Most chemotherapy given in the doctor's office flows into your blood in less than an hour. The kind of needle commonly used is a very thin metal needle, often called a "butterfly needle." It gets its name because the tabs on the side that the nurse holds onto during insertion look like the wings of a butterfly. Once the needle is in place, the wings are taped down to hold it still.

Right after insertion, you might see a little bit of blood flow back into the tubing attached to the needle. This indicates that the needle is inside the vein. Your nurse also verifies the correct placement of the IV by injecting a small amount of fluid into the needle. She or he can see that the fluid goes into the vein and not into the surrounding tissue. This shouldn't be painful, and once the needle is inserted and immobilized with tape there should be no further discomfort. Pain, burning, or swelling are all indications that the needle may not be in the vein or that the vein is leaking. You should tell your nurse immediately if you are having any of these symptoms.

Once the needle is secured and its position is verified, the medication will be given. It might be given through a syringe directly into the tubing of the butterfly needle. Or it may be diluted with a small amount of fluid from a bottle or plastic bag and dripped through tubing into your vein over a longer period of time. Once again, there should be no pain once the needle is secured.

Longer-Term IVs

If your treatment requires you to have an IV in your arm for a number of hours or longer, you need to be able to move around without dislodging the needle or damaging the vein. For longer term IVs, a thin, soft tube called an *IV catheter* is used. The catheter is about an inch long. At first, the catheter covers a thin steel needle. Once the catheter and needle are inserted into the vein, the steel needle is removed, leaving the soft, flexible catheter in place. The catheter is then secured by tape and a small dressing or bandage is put over the place where the catheter enters your skin. This catheter may stay in place for up to three days, but it may need to be changed sooner if there is any pain, swelling, redness, or signs of infection.

As with the steel butterfly needle, the position in the vein is verified by the presence of blood in the tubing and by having a small amount of fluid rinsed through the catheter into the vein without causing pain or swelling of the surrounding tissue.

How Do You Cope?

Most nurses who work with chemotherapy have a lot of experience in starting IVs and are very skillful as well as relaxed and supportive. They know that most of their patients are anxious, especially when first getting chemotherapy. You are not the only one who feels this way.

People have different ways of coping with stressful situations. Some people cope by learning everything they can about a new experience. It helps them if they know what will happen, what it will look like, what it will feel like, and what will be expected of them. Others cope by withdrawing into themselves. They don't want a lot of detailed information, since it just makes them feel overwhelmed and more anxious. Distraction helps other people. They feel more relaxed if they can focus on something else—meditation, reading, watching TV, or talking.

Many people say it helps to have a close friend or relative with them for support. The support can be both physical (holding their hand, for instance) and emotional. Having someone to talk to you, distract you, read to you, or just sit quietly with you can make you feel safer and more comfortable in a stressful situation. If you do bring along a support person, be sure that the person knows what you want from him or her. Talk it over and be specific about what will help you. Do you want a quiet, calm presence, or would you rather have someone distract you with conversation and gossip?

Take some time to think about how you cope with stress—and then do all the things you can to support your coping style. Would it help you to be familiar with the environment? You can arrange to meet the nurses, see the room where chemotherapy is given, and see other patients who are receiving treatment. The nurses can tell you exactly what to expect and how long the process takes and give you answers to many questions.

While you are getting chemotherapy, your nurses can also be a source of support. Don't forget to communicate how they can help. Let them know what your needs are. You might say, "It would help me to know exactly what I can expect. Please explain everything that is happening." Or you might say, "I brought a tape with me so I can just space out." Or, "I'd like my brother to stay with me."

Get comfortable. Because chemotherapy patients often have to sit still for an extended period of time, most clinics have comfortable recliner chairs or beds for them. Loosen tight waistbands, ties, or collars. Bring a sweater or shawl or ask your nurse for a warm blanket if you get cold. Try to position the arm that has the IV comfortably. Since some chemotherapy medicines leave a metallic taste in your mouth (or your mouth may feel dry from antinausea drugs or from anxiety), sucking on hard candy or chewing gum can be a help. The antinausea medications that you may get before your chemotherapy can also make you sleepy. If you feel that way, you may want to doze or listen to music on tape. Some clinics provide audio or video tapes or have a television that you can watch. Feel free to bring in your own tapes as well.

After your first treatment, your anxiety level should be much lower. The whole procedure, the environment, and the physical experience will be a little more familiar. You will also know more about what works and doesn't work to help you relax. Were you able to meditate, or was the room too distracting? Did your sister's endless chatter help pass the time, or was it annoying? Should you bring that murder mystery to read, or would you have preferred leafing through *People* magazine? You will also know the nurses better and feel more confident about their skill. And they will know you better and can begin to anticipate some of your individual physical and emotional needs.

Bags, Bottles, Tubing, and Pumps

IV fluids and medications flow through sterile tubing from a plastic bag or glass bottle. IVs flow by gravity, and the rate is adjusted with a roller clamp on the tube which controls the flow of fluid.

When the fluid or medicine needs to go at a set rate, it can be controlled with a special machine called an IV pump. An IV pump can be set at any rate. It also keeps track of how much fluid is left in the bag or bottle and can sense whether there is any resistance to the flow. Resistance may indicate that the needle is dislodged or the tubing is kinked. The pump also keeps an electronic eye out for any air bubbles in the tubing, and it will make a loud beep to alert you and your nurse if there is a problem. The IV pump is attached to the pole holding the medicines and fluids. The pump plugs into an electrical outlet, but it has a built-in battery so that it can be unplugged for short periods of time and still continue to function.

Sometimes two different bags or bottles of fluid will be running simultaneously in an IV. For instance, you might have a hydrating solution which provides water, a small amount of sugar, salts, and minerals. Another bag contains your chemotherapy, which is set to go in at a controlled rate over several hours or more. In addition, other bags might hold one or two IV medications to prevent nausea. These may be given both before your chemotherapy and at set intervals during your treatment. There may be times when your IV pole looks like a maze of bottles, tubes, and blinking lights, and you're not sure what is supposed to be dripping!

Some chemotherapy medicines are given very slowly—over several days. If you received this type of treatment, it used to require that you stay in the hospital for the duration of the treatment, although you may not really need hospital care. Now there are small portable IV pumps that are about the size of a small transistor radio or a paperback book. These pumps run on batteries, and are programmed by the nurses to deliver the IV medication at the prescribed rate. You can carry the pump with you in a bag, either over your shoulder or around your waist. That way you can be independent of poles, electrical outlets, and the hospital while getting treatment. The pump is equipped with an alarm to alert you if there is a problem with the machine or the flow of medication. If you get chemotherapy at home, you will probably be monitored by a visiting home-care nurse who specializes in IV therapy. You will be told how to contact the nurse, clinic, or hospital if problems arise, and to have the IV disconnected after the infusion is complete.

Your nurses will let you know what medicines you are getting, what they are for, and how they are likely to make you feel. For instance, some chemotherapy medicines are given with lots of hydrating fluids, and they will cause you to urinate frequently. Some antinausea medicines will make you feel sleepy or forgetful for a few hours. Knowing what to expect will make it all less frightening.

Staying Comfortable during Chemotherapy

During chemotherapy you should feel no pain or burning. Pain or burning from the IV may indicate that the needle or catheter is not positioned properly in the vein and that it should be checked or changed. You should not feel nauseated, because you will probably be given medicines to prevent nausea. Most people get through their chemotherapy treatments without any discomfort, continuing to eat and drink normally. Chapter 5 ("Coping with Nausea") will give you more information about the antinausea medicines and provide many self-help tips to avoid this problem.

Staying comfortable in part depends on you. Only you can tell how you feel. You are the source of the essential information about what's happening inside your body. If you have nausea, stomach cramps, dizziness, or any other unusual symptom, let your nurses know so that they can contact your doctor and have the medicines changed. It might take some fine-tuning to get you the medications and doses that will keep you comfortable, but it can and should be done.

IV Problems

It is the moment that everyone fears. Your veins are small, fragile, or invisible. You endure several attempts at starting the IV, and both you and the nurse get more and more tense. What should you do?

Go for the pro. Successfully starting an IV depends a great deal on the skill and experience of the person doing it. And generally the most skillful people are the ones who do it frequently.

In many hospitals there are special IV teams—nurses who are IV specialists. If you know that you are a "difficult start," you can ask for the IV specialist to see you, or you can ask for the most experienced nurse working on your floor or in the clinic. In time you will recognize some of the nurses and have more confidence in their ability. Just seeing a familiar face can help you relax, which helps your veins relax as well.

Stay calm. You have probably noticed that when you're anxious, your hands become cold and clammy. That's a normal reaction to fear. Unfortunately, anxiety works against you when you want the veins in your hands and arms to stand out. So anything you can do to lower your anxiety will probably help: deep breathing, having a supportive person with you, meditation, or even just a distraction. See Chapter 13 ("Relaxation and Stress Reduction") for more techniques.

Keep warm. Heat causes veins to dilate and fill with blood. That makes starting the IV easier. Your nurse may provide some form of heat for your arms, such as a warm blanket, heating pad, or a pan of warm water.

Keep drinking. Some people, afraid that they'll feel nauseated from their chemotherapy, don't eat or drink before their treatment. Since today's antinausea medications are so successful in preventing nausea, this really is not necessary. In fact, eating and drinking normally will keep your body fluids up and help make your IV easier to start. Your veins will be "fatter" (filled with more blood) if you don't let yourself become dehydrated.

What If Your IV Is Painful?

Sometimes, even if you've been careful not to disturb your IV, the catheter may become dislodged. Then the fluid or medicine, instead of flowing into your bloodstream, begins leaking into the tissue surrounding the vein. The affected area of your arm or hand might start to feel painful, tender, tight, or swollen. You may notice that your rings or watch feel tighter than usual. What should you do?

If you suspect that fluid is leaking out of the vein into the surrounding area, let your nurse know right away. It doesn't matter if it's day or night. The sooner the IV is removed and changed to another vein, the better. In the doctor's office, clinic, or hospital, the nurse will be watching your vein and the flow of fluid carefully, especially if the chemotherapy medicine is being injected directly into the tubing connected to the needle. Your nurse will check the flow of fluid as well as your arm and vein frequently. She or he will ask you if you have pain at the IV needle site. But don't wait to be asked. If you think there is swelling or if you have any discomfort, then call right away.

If you are getting IV fluids at home, call the visiting nursing or IV home-care agency (they should have someone available twenty-four hours a day) so they can advise you what to do immediately. They will send a nurse to evaluate the problem and restart the IV, if necessary.

Even if the catheter or needle is still in place and your vein is not leaking, your vein may feel irritated. Sometimes diluting the medicine with more fluid or slowing down the rate of the flow will help. Often, however, it is necessary for the nurse to change the IV to another vein (larger, if possible) so that the medicine can be swept along with a faster blood flow.

Monitoring the IV is clearly an important part of your treatment— and your nurse may not always be the first one to notice something. Even though she or he will often check your veins and the flow of medicine, it is always helpful for you to stay tuned in on your end.

Venous Access Devices

Figure 1 shows the veins of the arms and upper chest. The arm veins are called peripheral veins, and the blood flow through them is relatively slow compared to the larger veins of the upper chest. All peripheral veins lead to larger and larger veins, which carry a faster blood flow on the way to the heart. Chemotherapy treatments often involve multiple needle sticks for both blood tests and IVs and can become especially problematic if your arm veins are fragile or small.

Fortunately, new products have been developed to overcome some of these IV problems. The new products are called *venous access devices* (VAD). They provide a way into the larger veins of the blood system, where the blood moves more quickly and the effects of medicines and fluid are not as irritating. Venous access devices eliminate the difficulty of trying to find veins, and they make the process of starting IVs or taking blood tests quick and in some cases painless. They can also stay in place indefinitely, without interfering in your normal life at home.

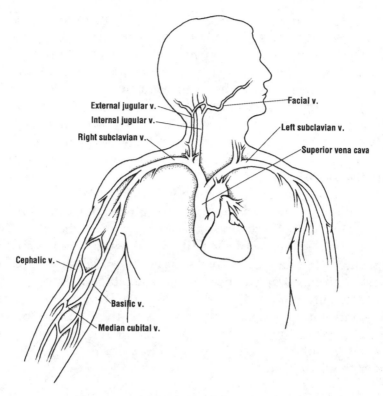

Figure 1   Veins of the Arms and Chest

Central Lines

Central IV catheters are inserted into one of the large veins in the upper chest. They are called central IV lines because they go into the veins nearer the heart. They may be used for longer-term treatments when the veins in the hands and arms are fragile or difficult to find or if the kind of IV fluids needed would be damaging to the smaller peripheral veins. The catheter can carry fluid, blood, chemotherapy, or other medicines, as well as provide blood for most blood tests.

This kind of catheter (shown in Figure 2) is inserted by a physician right in your hospital room or clinic, using a local anesthetic. Usually the catheter emerges from the skin near the collar bone where it is sutured into place. Because the place where the catheter emerges from the skin is so close to where the catheter penetrates the large vein, there is a risk of infection entering the bloodstream. Therefore the area where the catheter emerges must be kept sterile, and this requires special cleaning and dressings.

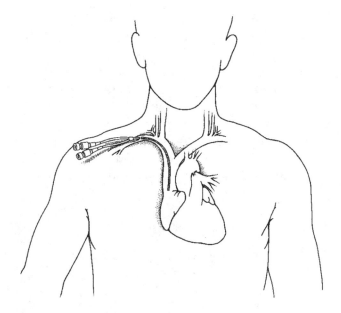

Figure 2   A Central IV Catheter

Although there is only one tiny hole in your skin where the catheter emerges, the end of the catheter may split into two or more ends or *lumens*. The fluid going into one lumen does not mix with the fluid going into the other lumen. This arrangement enables someone to administer more than one medication at the same time if necessary.

If you have this kind of catheter you will be given instructions and supplies to care for it at home. Your nurse at the clinic or the visiting nurses will be checking the skin around the catheter and changing the dressing. You will be taught how to change the caps as well as rinse the lumens with a special fluid to prevent a clot from forming inside the catheter.

Tunneled Catheters

These IV lines enter a big vein in your upper body, usually near the collar bone. The catheter is advanced until the end of the catheter is situated near the heart, where the blood flow is fastest. When a tunneled catheter is inserted, the physician makes a small incision near your collar bone and threads the catheter into a large central vein. Then he or she makes a tunnel under your skin from the vein towards the center of your chest. The catheter emerges from the front of your chest, at about the level of a second or third shirt button. Once the incision is healed and the minor swelling goes away, you should have no pain from the tunneled catheter. Figure 3 shows approximately where the catheter comes out of your body. Its position makes it easier to care for the skin around the catheter. You can clean the area yourself, and the little dressing doesn't show with your clothes on. Because the place where the catheter enters the vein (up by your collar bone) is far away from where it emerges from your skin (midchest), there is less chance of the large vein getting infected.

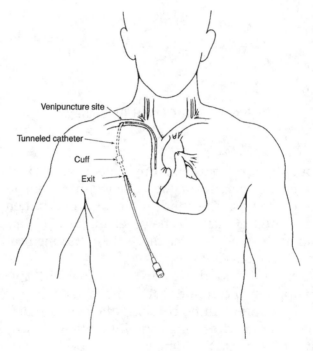

Figure 3   A Tunneled Catheter

A tunneled catheter means fewer needle sticks. The end of each lumen is capped off with a cap or rubber stopper. When the IV is started or a blood test is taken, the cap may be removed and the lumen is attached to an IV line or to a syringe to draw blood.

To prevent an infection, the tunneled catheter will require daily cleaning at the place where the catheter comes out of your skin, and each lumen must be routinely rinsed with special fluid to prevent a blood clot from forming. Your nurse will explain how and when to change the dressing and how to rinse the lumens and change the caps.

Implanted Vascular Access Devices

These catheters are also inserted into the large blood vessels of the upper chest. However, instead of emerging from the front of your chest, the catheter ends in a special device called a *port* that is implanted inside your skin (usually near your shoulder). Figure 4 shows an implanted port. The port is about the size of a half-dollar, and the raised center area is about the size of a nickel. The center area consists of a thick, rubberlike plug that can be punctured with a special needle that is usually attached to a short piece of IV tubing. Now the IV fluid, blood, or chemotherapy can flow into the port and through the catheter to the large veins.

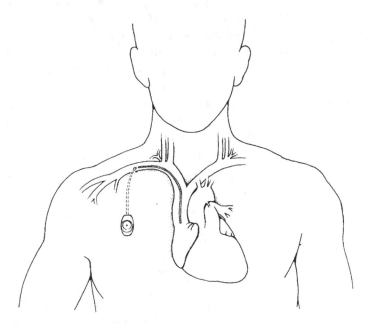

Figure 4   An Implanted Port

When you first need to have an IV started or blood drawn, the nurse feels for the location of the raised center of the port, cleans the skin, and punctures through the skin straight into the center plug. Since the center is usually easy to feel, there should be no fishing around as there often is with peripheral IVs. Success is not dependent on your veins. The needle is held securely by the center plug and is much less likely to be dislodged. Once the needle is inserted and secured, the port can be used for all fluids, IV medications, or blood. Most blood tests can be drawn from the same port and needle without any other needle sticks. When your treatment is finished, the catheter is rinsed with a solution that will prevent a clot from forming, and the needle is removed. If you need IV fluid over many days, the needle can stay in place under a sterile dressing for several days before the needle needs changing. When the needle is removed, the port under your skin automatically seals itself so there is none of the bleeding from the large vein that can sometimes happen after a blood test from a vein in your arm.

The implanted port and catheter are put in by a physician during a minor surgical procedure. The doctor makes a small incision below your collar bone, threads the catheter into the large vein, and then forms a little pocket for the port under the skin of your upper chest. Once the incision is healed and the tenderness and minor swelling go away, you should have no pain from the implanted port. Although you'll be able to feel the raised rubber center of the port, no part of the device is left outside of your skin. Once the incision is healed, you can bathe and even swim. No daily care is required, because your own skin protects the catheter from infection.

The implanted port and catheter can stay in place indefinitely and enable you to have most blood tests, IVs, and medications with only one needle stick.

Other IV Alternatives

New devices and techniques are always being developed to make the IV experience less traumatic, less painful, and more dependable. An alternative method for getting to the big veins uses a very long catheter that is inserted in an arm vein and then threaded up until it gets to the larger vein in the upper chest. This device (shown in Figure 5) is called a *peripheral inserted central catheter* (PICC) because the catheter is inserted peripherally (into your arm), but travels to a large central vein (in your chest). The end of the catheter emerges from your arm and requires special cleaning and dressings to prevent infection, similar to the central IV catheter described above.

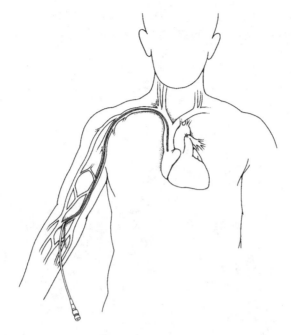

Figure 5   A Peripheral Inserted Central Catheter (PICC)

There is also a small port (shown in Figure 6) that can be implanted in your arm. As with the PICC, a long catheter then travels from your arm into a large vein of your upper chest. The advantage of this device over the PICC is that the catheter never emerges from your skin. It ends at the implanted port and remains sterile. It requires no special cleaning or dressing and, like the implanted chest port, needs only a single needle stick to gain access to the blood system.

Which One Is Right for You?

Not everyone will need a central line, tunneled catheter, or an implanted port. There are many, many people who complete their chemotherapy treatment and blood tests without needing any such device. Their veins can tolerate the kind of medications and fluid they need. Although it's never pleasant to have IVs started or blood drawn, they get through it without major problems.

If you need a venous access device, you and your doctor and nurse will discuss the risks and benefits of each one. Your doctor will consider the kind of chemotherapy you need, your anatomy, and your preference. You will be able to see what each device looks like and perhaps talk to someone who has one.

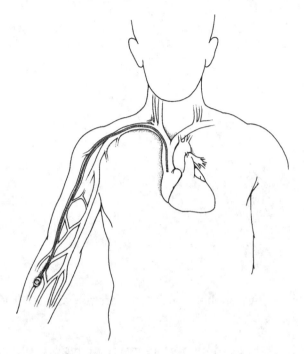

Figure 6   A Peripheral Implanted Port

Although it's not easy to face the minor surgery that's needed to have a VAD put in your body, once it is in place many people experience it as a great relief. Their IVs are easily started, blood tests are easily obtained, and their arms and hands are freer while they are getting treatment.

Getting Through It

For many people, a good deal of dread and fear about getting chemotherapy is associated with the frequent blood tests and IVs. They may feel out of control when their veins won't cooperate and having an IV started becomes difficult.

In time you'll find your own unique ways of relaxing and coping during this stressful period. Hopefully, you'll come to trust the skill and support of the people who are caring for you. Just knowing what to expect, what is happening, and what it will feel like can make it all less overwhelming.

5

Coping with Nausea

Of the possible side effects of cancer treatments, people often say they dread feeling nauseated and vomiting the most. They may have known someone who received chemotherapy or radiation therapy and who suffered severe nausea without effective antinausea medication. Or, they may recall times during their own lives when they were nauseated and remember how debilitating it was.

It's a misconception that people who receive cancer-fighting treatments such as chemotherapy and radiation therapy suffer continuous, unrelieved nausea and vomiting. First, it is important to remember that not all cancer-fighting treatments cause severe nausea. Some may cause mild nausea or no nausea at all. Second, nausea caused by chemotherapy or radiation therapy usually lasts for a limited amount of time (from two to forty-eight hours for most chemotherapy drugs, or for a few hours after radiation). Third, extensive research has led to the development of new medications that can prevent or relieve the nausea associated with cancer treatments.

What Causes Nausea?

The feeling of nausea and the act of vomiting are not really caused by your stomach. There is actually an area in your brain that, when stimulated, causes these feelings. It is called the *chemoreceptor trigger zone* (CTZ), and it lies in the center of your brain. This area may be stimulated by a number of different events. The CTZ may be simulated by a feeling of fullness in your stomach (from too much pizza and beer, for example), or it may be stimulated by dizziness (sea sickness or motion sickness). Certain sights, smells, or thoughts may cause nausea as well. Some people may feel nauseated and even vomit from anxiety, fear, stage fright, the sight of blood, unpleasant smells, or the thought of getting an injection.

Nausea and Chemotherapy

The CTZ is sensitive to the chemicals in your body. Some chemotherapy drugs make your body release other chemicals, such as dopamine or seratonin, which can stimulate the CTZ. Every chemotherapy drug has been rated as to its *emetic potential*—the chances that it will cause you to feel nauseated or to vomit. Some drugs rarely cause nausea (meaning that less than 30 percent of people taking the drug feel that symptom). Some are considered only moderately nauseating. And then there are drugs that are very likely to make you feel nauseated, meaning that 90 percent of the people report the symptom. So, right from the beginning, your doctor can tell you if nausea is likely to be a problem.

Another factor that may determine how nauseated you feel is the dose. A chemotherapy drug may not cause nausea at a low dose, but it may cause the problem at higher doses or when given in combination with other more nauseating drugs.

Nausea and Radiation Therapy

Nausea can be a problem if radiation therapy is directed to your digestive system. Sometimes the radiation is not directly focused on the digestive system, but it may be exposed to radiation if other nearby structures are being radiated. For instance, radiation to lymph nodes in the abdomen can cause nausea when the stomach or intestines come within the radiation field. Nausea can also be a problem when radiation treatments cause a decrease in the normal amount of stomach secretions, or change how the small intestines absorb fluids. The CTZ can also be stimulated by waste products (created by the destruction of tumor cells), or more directly, when the brain itself is radiated.

There are always individual differences in how people react to any treatment. Some people are just more likely to feel nauseated, just as there are some people who are more likely to suffer morning sickness or motion sickness. Your doctor may try to predict how much of a problem nausea will be, but you may be less or more nauseated than expected. The key is to work with your doctor and nurse to determine the type and the amount of antinausea medication you need to prevent or minimize the problem.

Types of Antinausea Medicines and How They Work

The stimulus that triggers nausea can come from different places in your body—from the stomach, the inner ear, even from sensations and thoughts, as well as from chemicals or radiation. To prevent or relieve nausea, different drugs work in different ways. Some drugs prevent nausea by blocking the body's release of histamine, dopamine, or serotonin, so that the CTZ will not be stimulated. Some drugs speed up the stomach and intestines to make the stomach empty quickly so that there is less fullness to stimulate the CTZ. Some drugs block or neutralize stomach acids. Other medications help you relax and even sleep through the period of time when you are most likely to feel nauseated.

Keep in mind that whether or not you become nauseated from chemotherapy or radiation does not indicate if the treatments are working. And when you get medications to prevent or relieve the nausea, it does not make the treatments less effective.

The following group of drugs is commonly used to prevent nausea during chemotherapy and radiation treatments. The generic name is given first, followed by the brand name(s) that may be more familiar to you. Next comes a general discussion of how the drug works, and some side effects to watch out for.

Prochlorperazine (Compazine®). This drug has been the mainstay of antinausea treatment for over thirty years. It acts in the CTZ by blocking dopamine receptors. Dopamine is released by the body in response to some chemotherapy drugs and can cause nausea. Compazine can be used alone for preventing nausea when you are getting mildly nauseating chemotherapy or radiation treatments. It is available in many forms, including a pill, a long-acting capsule, a rectal suppository, an injection in the muscle, or by IV.

Side effects to watch for are drowsiness (don't drive) and low blood pressure (usually only a problem if given by IV). Compazine may also cause an uncomfortable jittery feeling or restlessness. This reaction is called *akathesia* and it goes away if you take a mild tranquilizer such as diazepam (Valium®), or lorazepam (Ativan®). You may also experience a tightness in the muscles of your jaw or face. This is called *dystonia* and is easily relieved by taking a mild antihistamine, such as diphenhydramine (Benadryl®), which is available from the drugstore without a prescription. If you are having any of these side effects, be sure to call your doctor to see if he or she wants you to change to a different medication or to take additional medications to counteract these symptoms.

Lorazepam (Ativan®). This drug is a tranquilizer in the same family as Valium. It doesn't block dopamine at the CTZ or speed up the digestive tract, but works by making you relaxed, forgetful, and sleepy. It is sometimes used alone, but often in combination with other antinausea drugs when patients are getting moderately to highly nauseating chemotherapy or radiation therapy. You can take this drug by mouth, by injection in the muscle, or by IV. Only the nongeneric (brand name) form of this drug (Ativan®) is easily absorbed under the tongue through the mucous membranes. This is particularly helpful if you are vomiting or having difficulty getting pills down.

The side effects to watch for are sedation and forgetfulness. Do not drive when taking this drug. You may find that you do not remember events or conversations you have had while taking lorazepam. It may also cause unsteadiness, weakness, or a mild lowering of blood pressure. Call your doctor if these side effects are a problem. You may need to use a smaller dose, take it less often, or change to a different medication. Taken at night, lorazepam can help you fall asleep, as well as relieve nausea.

Ondansetron (Zofran®). This relatively new antinausea drug has been used since 1991. It works by preventing serotonin (a chemical released by your body in response to chemotherapy or radiation therapy) from getting through to the CTZ and causing nausea. Zofran is very effective in preventing nausea from even the most nauseating cancer-fighting treatments. It is sometimes given by IV right before chemotherapy and again after four and eight hours. It is also effective at a higher dose given just once prior to chemotherapy, and the effect will last for about twenty-four hours. If nausea lasts longer than twenty-four hours, Zofran can be repeated daily for the next few days as well, although it seems to work better during the early phase of nausea. Zofran is now available as a pill that you can take every eight to twelve hours to relieve nausea at home after radiation therapy or chemotherapy.

One advantage of Zofran is that it does not have the side effects of some of the other antinausea medicines. It will not make you sleepy, and does not cause the restlessness or muscle stiffness that prochlorperazine (Compazine) has been known to cause. One possible side effect of Zofran is constipation. To prevent this problem you should increase your fluids and take a stool softener on the days you are using this drug. You may also need to take a laxative if you don't have a bowel movement after a day or so. Zofran can also cause a mild headache. Ask your doctor or nurse for a pain reliever if you are having this symptom.

Granisetron (Kytril®). Kytril is similar to Zofran. It works by preventing seratonin from getting through to the CTZ and causing nausea. Kytril is usually given once prior to chemotherapy to prevent nausea, and the antinausea effect lasts about twenty-four hours. Kytril is now available by pill and is taken twice a day to prevent nausea at home. Kytril does not cause sleepiness or muscle stiffness like Compazine, but like Zofran, it can cause constipation. Increase fluids and take a stool softener to prevent this problem, or use a laxative if neccessary. Kytril has also been known to cause headache, which can be relieved with a mild pain reliever.

Steroids (dexamethasone—Decadron®, Hexadrol®). It is not known exactly how steroids work to prevent nausea. It's possible that they prevent the chemicals that are released by the body in response to chemotherapy or radiation therapy from getting through to the CTZ, and therefore make it less likely that you will feel nauseated. This drug is available as a pill, but it is usually given by IV in combination with other antinausea drugs prior to treatment. For instance, you may get IV Decadron along with Zofran or Kytril.

Side effects to watch for are water retention, restlessness, confusion, insomnia, and euphoria (feeling high). Also, if it is given too rapidly by IV, steroids may cause a temporary feeling of itchiness or burning in the vaginal or rectal area, but this lasts only a few minutes and goes away on its own. People who have diabetes need to be aware that steroids can cause a temporary elevation in blood sugar. Steroids taken by pill can be irritating to the lining of the stomach, and that in itself can cause nausea. Always take steroid pills with food to prevent stomach irritation.

Combinations of drugs. As you can tell from the preceding list of medications, different antinausea drugs work in different ways. One drug prevents the chemicals that are released by your body in response to cancer-fighting treatment from affecting the CTZ. Another helps decrease anxiety, making you relaxed and sleepy. Some drugs prevent the immediate nausea associated with treatments, and others are effective in relieving nausea that can occur several days after treatment.

There are other drugs your doctor may use in combination with those listed above. For instance, antihistamines such as diphenyhydramine (Benadryl®) are useful in preventing nausea associated with motion sickness. When used with other antinausea medications, Benadryl can make them even more effective. Metoclopramide (Reglan®) helps the stomach empty quickly by speeding up the digestive tract. Smoking marijuana or taking the drug dronabinol (Marinol®) (which contains the active ingredient in marijuana) in combination with other antinausea medications can help prevent nausea, as well as stimulate your appetite. Drugs which neutralize or decrease stomach acid (Pepcid®, Prilosec®, Tagamet®, Zantac®, etc.) can also help to prevent or relieve nausea when used with other antinausea drugs.

Every medicine has potential side effects. To be safe, always consult with your doctor or nurse before taking any new medicines, even ones you can buy without a prescription.

How to Take Antinausea Medicines

Start by taking the medication in the dose and frequency recommended. For instance, your doctor might recommend taking Compazine every four to six hours. Be alert to any side effects that may occur, and notify your doctor or nurse as soon as possible if you are having any problems. Remember, everyone has his or her own unique responses to treatment, and to the antinausea medicines. Your doctor needs your feedback to make adjustments in the plan so that it works for you. You may need to change to a different medication. You may need to change the schedule, the dose, or frequency of the medication, or you may need to add another medication to counteract a bothersome side effect.

Nausea from Anticipation

You may develop nausea that is not directly caused by the chemotherapy or radiation. People who suffer unrelieved nausea from cancer treatments begin to automatically associate the treatments with feeling nauseated. This is a conditioned response to a strongly unpleasant experience. As a result, anything associated with the treatment may trigger this reaction—the ride to the office or hospital, the sight of the nurse, the IV tubing, the smell of alcohol, or entering the dressing room at the radiation therapy department. This phenomenon of feeling nauseated without a physical reason is called *anticipatory nausea and vomiting* (ANV). The best treatment for ANV is prevention. If you didn't suffer significant nausea with one treatment, then you are not likely to anticipate feeling nauseated with the next one.

Anxiety also contributes to anticipatory nausea. Some people avoid pretreatment jitters and nausea by taking antinausea medication even before they leave the house. Or, if they have to drive, they may take the pill immediately after arriving for their appointment. The medication that seems to work best for ANV is Ativan, but anything that allows you to relax can help prevent nausea. The following are a few suggestions.

Progressive muscle relaxation (PMR) is a way of counteracting anxiety. You can learn to relax all the muscles of your body, visualize pleasant scenes, and psychologically remove yourself from a stressful environment. See Chapter 13 ("Relaxation and Stress Reduction") for more information on PMR.

Systematic desensitization has been used successfully for this problem as well. This technique is a kind of counterconditioning used in the treatment of anxiety and phobia. After you learn to relax your body, various anxiety-provoking scenes associated with chemotherapy are visualized, starting from the least anxiety-provoking to the most. For instance, you might start by visualizing driving to the clinic or doctor's office for your treatment. You learn to relax while visualizing this scene. Then you slowly work up to the scarier scenes (such as having the IV started, or lying on the radiation treatment table). When you learn to relax your body while visualizing the whole procedure from beginning to end, you may find that you are less anxious and less nauseated.

In addition to PMR and systematic desensitization, other relaxation techniques may prove useful in relieving anticipatory nausea, and are explained in Chapter 13. Deep breathing, relaxation imagery, autogenics, and self-hypnosis are excellent ways to relax. Sometimes just bringing a book or magazine to glance through may distract you. Some people find that bringing a friend to sit and chat, or listening to some music with headphones, is helpful to lower their anxiety and lessen their chances of anticipatory nausea.

The Importance of Fluid

Everything that you take by mouth (food, fluid, medication, and so on) eventually enters your bloodstream, where it circulates through your entire body. It is finally removed from the blood by the liver or kidneys and is eliminated in the urine. Some chemotherapy drugs can cause direct damage to the bladder or kidneys if they are not eliminated fast enough. Dying tumor cells release chemical waste products after chemotherapy or radiation therapy, which can cause nausea. That is why it is so important to drink plenty of fluid after your treatments. The more fluid you take in, the easier it is for your body to break down the chemical by-products and eliminate them.

One of the dangers of continuous nausea and vomiting is that it makes if difficult to take fluids by mouth. When you are in the hospital or clinic, you will probably receive fluids directly into your bloodstream by IV. But when you are home, after your treatment or after a stay in the hospital, it is especially important to control nausea so that you can drink. If you are too nauseated to drink, you may become dry or dehydrated. When you are dry, the nausea may get worse. The result is a vicious cycle: unrelieved nausea causes dehydration, which intensifies the nausea. Preventing that cycle is essential.

What Is Dehydration?

If you have not been able to drink because of nausea, or if you've been vomiting a great deal, you will feel dry. Your mouth and lips will be dry and may be flaky or cracked. Your blood pressure may be lower than usual, and so you may feel dizzy when first standing up. (Note that since some antinausea medicines can cause dry mouth and slight dizziness, those symptoms may not necessarily mean that you are dehydrated.) When you are dehydrated your body will try to hold onto all the fluid it can, so you will notice that you are urinating less frequently and that the volume of urine is less than usual. Your urine may appear darker because it is more concentrated. You may notice that your weight is down several pounds from before you had your treatment. These are all signs of dehydration.

Preventing Dehydration

Here are some suggestions for the hours after your treatment to prevent dehydration:

1. When you first get home, take the antinausea medication at the dose and time recommended. Take it before you experience nausea. That way you can continue to take fluids and eliminate the byproducts of treatment—and feel better sooner.

2. Follow the set schedule of medications as recommended by your doctor or nurse. That will keep you covered during the hours when you're most likely to have problems.

3. If your nausea is not relieved by the medication, or you're having problems with side effects, contact your doctor or nurse. They may advise you to change the dose or frequency of the medication, or add another medication that will relieve your symptoms or counteract side effects. You might need to take a medication by rectal suppository until you're able to keep fluid down.

What to Do If You Are Becoming Dehydrated

Be sure that you are taking the antinausea medication prescribed. If you are vomiting and cannot keep pills down, call your doctor for advice. After taking the medication, wait about half an hour and then try sips of fluid. Any kind of fluid is fine—water, tea, popsicles, or broth. Drink a small amount frequently (try half a cup every half hour). At first you may only be able to tolerate water, but once you feel a little better, try drinking fluids that have calories, such as soda, diluted fruit juice, popsicles, tea with honey, etc. You need some calories or you will feel very weak. Add easily digested solid food cautiously. You may be able to tolerate a little sherbet, applesauce, or toast. See Chapter 7 ("Maintaining Good Nutrition") for more suggestions on how and what to eat when coping with nausea.

Keep track of how much fluid you are taking and how often you are vomiting, as well as how often you are urinating. If you are still nauseated and think you may be getting dehydrated, call your doctor. Don't wait until you are severely dehydrated to call. Be sure to supply the kind of information that will enable your doctor to accurately evaluate your condition. Tell the doctor:

1. How much fluid you drank in the last twenty-four hours

2. How often and approximately how much you have vomited in the last twenty-four hours

3. What antinausea medicines have been prescribed, whether or not you have taken them, and what problems, if any, they have caused

4. How often and approximately how much you have urinated, and if your urine appears dark. (Some chemotherapy medicines will discolor your urine for a few hours, so it may be difficult to tell if your urine appears darker than normal due to dehydration.)

5. If you have lost weight since getting your treatment (weigh yourself before you call)

6. If your mouth, lips, and skin feel dry

7. If and when you feel dizzy. (Does it happen all the time or just when first rising from a sitting or lying position?)

8. If you have other symptoms that are affecting your condition, such as:

    If you have a fever (take your temperature before calling)

    If you have pain—where, how long it lasts, what makes it better or worse

    If you are diabetic (check your blood sugar before calling)

    If you have missed taking other medications because of the nausea or vomiting (heart or blood pressure medication, anticonvulsants, pain medication, hormones, steroids, etc.)

If you have other digestion problems such as diarrhea heart burn, bloating, etc.

Your doctor may want you to come into the office or clinic to check your blood pressure and test your blood to see how dehydrated you may have become. It may be necessary to give you extra fluid and antinausea medications by IV as well as to make changes in the medications you take at home. Dehydration is a temporary condition that is usually corrected quickly with replaced fluids and medicines.

Step-by-Step Hints

Before Treatment

It is not necessary to have an empty stomach before getting chemotherapy or radiation therapy. Staying well nourished and well hydrated (drinking lots of fluids) will help you feel stronger and help your body eliminate waste products more quickly. Eat and drink regularly until about two hours before your treatment. Eat foods that are easily digested (high carbohydrate, low fat). Stay away from spicy food or food that will give you a lingering aftertaste that may make you feel nauseated later (onions, garlic, etc.). Your doctor may want you to take antinausea medicine before coming to the clinic or hospital.

During Treatment

Do whatever you can to lower your anxiety. Bring a book, a music tape, or a friend to occupy you while you are waiting for treatment. Some antinausea medicine might make you feel sleepy, so sleeping through longer chemotherapy treatments might be possible. Wear comfortable clothes, loosen your belt or tie, and bring a sweater or ask for a blanket if you feel cold. Some chemotherapy drugs leave a metallic or unpleasant taste in your mouth, so sucking on hard candy or chewing gum might help.

After Treatment

Medications. Take the antinausea medications as prescribed. Do not wait to feel nauseated to take the medications. Your aim is to get through the high-risk hours and not feel nauseated at all.

Food and Fluids. Eat small amounts, more frequently. Avoid feeling overfull. Eat bland foods (mashed potatoes, cottage cheese, toast, sherbet, crackers).

You may be very sensitive to smells of food. Foods that are served cold or at room temperature have less aroma. Stay out of the kitchen as mush as possible. Prepare foods for yourself or the family that are quick and easy with minimal sights or smells that may be upsetting to you.

If you are diabetic, you have to be careful that the medication you take to control your blood sugar is appropriate for how much you are eating. You might need to check your blood sugar several times on the day of your treatment to make sure it is not getting too low or too high. Your doctor may want to adjust your insulin dose or other blood sugar medication until you're able to eat normally.

Sometimes sweet juices are hard to tolerate after treatment. If that's true for you, try lemonade, broth, club soda, or ice water. Try mixing a little juice with mineral water. You might need to try several different kinds of tastes before you discover what works best.

It is most important to take fluids. Don't worry if at first you don't feel like eating solid foods. Try popsicles, tea, juices, soup, soda, or ice. Drinking with your meal may make you feel overfull and bloated, so drink fluids before or after eating solid food. Drink small amounts of fluids frequently to avoid feeling too full.

Rinse your mouth or brush your teeth before and after eating to avoid lingering tastes that may be nauseating.

Activities. Fresh air and mild physical activity help prevent nausea. Take a walk or sit on the porch or by an open window. Distractions may help. Go to the movies, read a book, talk to a friend, listen to music, play cards, and so on.

Sleep. Some antinausea medications may make you sleepy. Let yourself sleep through the high-risk hours. If you are supposed to take some medication on a set schedule around the clock, you may want to set the alarm clock so that you can wake up, take the medication, and then go back to sleep. If you are not taking antinausea medication in the middle of the night, then take it when you first wake up—before you get out of bed and start moving around.

Relaxation. If you are feeling anxious, relaxing may be easier said than done. There are a number of audio and video tapes that you may find useful to help you clear your mind and relax every muscle in your body. You may find that the tension you are holding in your face and jaw or in your shoulders or abdominal muscles is adding to your anxiety or feelings of queasiness. Some tapes provide peaceful and relaxing images and music. After you practice with these tapes for a period of time, you may be able to relax yourself very quickly with or without the tape any time you feel tense or anxious. You can also make your own tape with the relaxation scripts provided in Chapter 14 at the end of this book.

Self-Talk. The things you say to yourself can either help you cope or cause you more stress. Many of these thoughts are unconscious and so automatic that you may not even be aware of them Pay attention and try to tune into what you may be saying to yourself that is increasing your stress and worries about nausea (or any other scary symptom). It may help to write these thoughts down. This makes them more conscious and more manageable. It also allows you to argue against them and replace these anxiety-provoking thoughts with thoughts that are supportive, accurate, and focused on coping. Your anxiety-producing thoughts may sound like this:

I can't stand it—this is too much.
I feel so helpless, there is nothing I can do.
The antinausea medicine isn't working—nothing will help.
I'll never feel any better.

You can replace these with supportive thoughts that help you cope:

I can get through this—the discomfort will only last a few hours.
If this medicine isn't working to relieve my nausea, there are other medicines that I can try.
The chemotherapy/radiation is effective, no matter how nauseated I feel.
I'm learning how my body reacts to chemotherapy/radiation and to the antinausea medicines.
I am in charge—I can take the medicine that I need in order to feel better.
It's okay to sleep and let the hours pass.
The kids (or husband, or job) are taken care of for now. Right now I can pay attention to me and take care of myself.

I know how to relax, distract myself, and feel better.

I know that _____ is here for me if I need him/her.

Write down your own coping thoughts. When you find your anxiety rising, tune into what you are silently saying to yourself and talk back, using the coping statements that help you feel better.

Nausea and vomiting can be very debilitating, both physically and emotionally. Fortunately, there are strong and effective medications and relaxation techniques that really work. Lots of people get through their chemotherapy treatment with minimal nausea or no nausea at all. That is the goal—to get through this time and remain comfortable, well nourished, and able to do the normal activities of your life as soon as possible. Preventing this side effect is very important. If you are able to stay well nourished, feel good, and maintain your activities, you will be more able and willing to complete your treatment. This is possible only if side effects like nausea and vomiting can be controlled.

6

Coping with Other Digestion Problems

When people think about the side effects of chemotherapy and radiation therapy, nausea and vomiting are the symptoms that most frequently come to mind. But other parts of the digestive system can be affected as well. Unlike nausea, which is associated with the period of time immediately following treatment, other digestive system side effects may not be apparent until a week or two later. Here's why.

Chemotherapy and radiation therapy affect cells that are frequently dividing—these include the cells lining your entire digestive system. Normally, cells that are old or dying are shed and replaced by new cells. But if there is a delay in the replacement of old cells because of the effects of chemotherapy or radiation therapy, then you can develop problems such as a sore mouth and throat, taste changes, and diarrhea or constipation. This chapter will discuss these and other side effects that can cause temporary changes in the digestive system, why they occur, and what you can do to feel better.

While chemotherapy travels through the blood system, potentially affecting every cell in the body and every part of the digestive system, radiation therapy affects only the part of the body that is exposed to the radiation. That includes the tumor itself and structures nearby that are within the radiation field. This means that radiation of lymph nodes in the abdomen may cause nausea or diarrhea, but will not cause mouth sores or taste changes. Your radiation oncologist and nurses will tell you what specific side effects can occur from the radiation treatments you are receiving, when you can expect them, and when they will go away. In general, side effects from radiation therapy develop slowly over the weeks of treatment, and they will slowly resolve after all the treatments are completed.

Parts of the Digestive System

In order to visualize the way food travels through your body, you might think of a large tube. This tube starts at your mouth and ends at your rectum. The mouth is the place where the digestion of food and fluids starts. When you chew, the food is mixed with saliva, which begins to break down the food into substances the body can use.

When you swallow, the food and fluids travel down a long, straight section of the tube called the *esophagus*, which connects to your stomach. Once in the stomach, food is further broken down by the mechanical action of muscles churning and the chemical action of the acidic digestive enzymes found there.

The partially digested food moves from your stomach into the small intestine, which is approximately twenty-one feet long. Because it's so long and the space in your abdomen is fairly compact, the intestine winds back and forth in your abdominal cavity like a ribbon. It is in the small intestine that most of the nutrients are absorbed into your bloodstream.

What remains of food after digestion are waste products. These move into the large intestine (also known as the colon). The colon is about five feet in length and ends with your rectum. As the waste products move through the large intestine, fluid is absorbed. By the time the waste products have traveled through the entire colon and are ready to be eliminated from your body, the stool is no longer liquid, but a formed solid.

Mouth and Throat Problems

During the months you are receiving cancer treatments (chemotherapy or radiation therapy treatments), there may be times when your mouth and throat become sore. The soreness may start with a feeling of hypersensitivity to sour or spicy tastes and some redness or swelling of your gums, cheeks, pallet, or throat. There may be open areas similar to cold sores on the sides. Brushing your teeth, rinsing with a mouthwash, eating, or even swallowing may be very painful.

Your doctor or nurse may call this condition *mucositis* or *stomatitis*. Mucositis means an inflammation of the mucous membranes of your gastrointestinal system, while stomatitis is an inflammation of the mucous linings of your mouth. Both terms describe the problems that may occur when the surface layer of cells lining your mouth and throat are not replaced as quickly as usual because of the chemotherapy or radiation therapy. If you have inflammation or sores in your esophagus, it's called *esophagitis*.

Radiation of the head or neck or chemotherapy agents such as 5-Fluorouracil (5-FU) are most likely to cause mouth sores. As with any side effect caused by cancer treatments, the chance of developing the problem and the severity of the problem are related not only to the type of medication or treatment, but also to the dose and your general health and age. Not everyone will develop mucositis, but it is good to be able to recognize the problem early and know what to do. While this condition is painful and uncomfortable, it will improve fairly quickly as the cells recuperate. However, during the time you are experiencing mucositis, there are a number of things that you can try to feel better, promote healing, and prevent infection.

Self-Help Suggestions for Mouth and Throat Sores

1. Keep your mouth clean and comfortable. First, the cleaner your mouth is, the better it will feel and the faster it will heal. Brushing your teeth or dentures and rinsing your mouth within thirty minutes after meals is very important. When your mouth is sore or your platelet count is low you need to be especially careful not to cause more irritation or bruising. Use a soft toothbrush. Wetting your toothbrush in hot water will soften the bristles even more. If your mouth is very sore, or your platelets are so low that gentle brushing causes bleeding, you can use a sponge-tipped swab to gently clean your mouth as well as to stimulate your mucous membranes. Although sponge-tipped swabs are not as effective as a tooth- brush in removing debris or plaque from your teeth, they can help you get your teeth cleaner than just a rinse. Go back to using your toothbrush when your mouth tissues heal and platelet count improves. If your platelet count is low, do not use floss or a strong stream of water from a "water-jet", as these could also cause bleeding.

Dentures and partials can cause some irritation to sensitive mouth tissues when they are sore, even if they fit well. It may be helpful to remove them while you are sleeping at night or for short periods during the day. Try to keep your lips moist by using a lip gel or even a light layer of Vaseline. Most lip gels or balms have an oil base which will protect your lips for several hours. Some brands have sunscreen in them as well. Soon you will notice that the dry skin is noticeably softer and that any cracks are beginning to heal.

2. Use a mouth rinse. In addition to using a tartar control toothpaste, rinse and gargle with a dilute solution of baking soda. Use one half-teaspoon of baking soda mixed into a half-cup of water. The baking soda solution cleans, promotes healing, and lowers the acidity in your mouth. This is especially helpful if you have vomited and some of the stomach acid has come up into your mouth. Rinsing with a baking-soda solution will help to neutralize the effects of acidic debris on your tender oral tissues.

If you have a sore mouth, avoid using commercial mouthwashes or products which contain alcohol or glycerin. Both will dry your mouth tissues even more and make the soreness worse.

3. Eating hints. When your mouth or throat is sore, avoid foods which are hot or spicy. Foods that contain chili powder or pepper (like some Mexican or Thai dishes) may cause more pain. Avoid drinks that are so hot that they make your mouth sting. Citrus juices (such as orange or grapefruit juices) may also be a problem because they are acidic. Cool, bland fluids (apple juice, grape juice, herbal teas) will be more soothing to your mouth and throat.

Mouth Pain

Most people are able to cope with the short period of time that their mouths and throats are sore without too much difficulty. But sometimes mouth pain is so severe that it interferes with your ability to eat or drink. When you have severe pain in other parts of your body, you would naturally try to protect that part by resting it until it was no longer hurting. When your mouth is sore, that remedy is not possible, since you must continue to take fluids and nourishment orally. One thing that may help is rinsing with a topical anesthetic (like the dentist uses before injections). This will temporarily relieve pain so you can eat or clean your mouth. But be aware that if you swallow the numbing medicine, it will also suppress your natural gag reflex. You must be careful when you swallow because, if the gag reflex is not working, food or liquid can more easily be swallowed the "wrong way."

If your mouth pain is so severe that you cannot eat or drink enough fluids to prevent dehydration, you may need to have IV fluids and pain medication for a few days until you are feeling better.

Taste Changes

After a time, some foods which previously tasted good to you may have a different, even unpleasant flavor. For example, red meat may taste bitter, or sweet foods may taste more or less sweet than you are used to. The reason for this is that your taste buds may be temporarily altered by the chemotherapy or radiation treatments. Even foods that you crave may taste different in an unpleasant way.

Taste changes are usually not permanent. Even after the high doses of chemotherapy given for bone marrow transplantation, people report that their sense of taste eventually returns to normal. But give it time; it may take several months. In the meantime, here are some ways you can deal with the problem.

Cleaning your mouth by brushing and rinsing with the baking soda solution (described above) before meals can help. When your mouth is clean and moist, flavors of foods may be more distinct. If your mouth feels like it is filled with cotton, the taste of food will not be as pleasant.

Experiment with eating foods that have various kinds of flavors to see which ones taste good to you and which ones to avoid. When your sense of taste is diminished or altered, try eating foods with different textures or temperatures to make a meal more interesting. Chapter 7 has more suggestions about how to deal with taste changes. A consultation with a nutritionist could be helpful in finding foods that are more appealing so you can stay well nourished even while you are experiencing this problem.

Yeast Infections

There is a normal balance of organisms that naturally live in and on your body. When this balance changes, you are more likely to develop a yeast infection. For example, many women know that when they are taking antibiotics they are more likely to develop vaginal yeast infections. The normal balance of organisms that live in your mouth can also be changed because of cancer treatments, medications, or a change in your nutrition. White patches on the insides of your cheeks, on your tongue, or along the gum line may indicate that you have a yeast infection in your mouth (also known as thrush). Call your doctor or nurse so that he or she can prescribe an antifungal medication (such as nystatin or Mycostatin) to eliminate the problem. These antifungal medicines come in lozenge or liquid form. Use them after eating, brushing, and rinsing, and do not rinse again for at least thirty minutes. In that way you can keep the medicine on the affected areas to promote healing.

If the medication comes as a lozenge, let it melt slowly in your mouth so that it can cover all your mouth surfaces as well as your throat. If you have difficulty with the lozenges because your mouth is very dry or sore, tell your doctor or nurse to order the medication in a liquid form.

When using the liquid, take about a teaspoon of it and swish it around in your mouth so that it covers all of the surfaces of your cheeks and gums. Then let it roll back into your throat and gargle with it so that it can also coat your throat. You can then either swallow it or spit it out. (Since your esophagus may also be sore or infected, swallowing the antifungal solution will allow it to coat and heal this area as well.)

Another way to take the antifungal solution is to measure out your doses into ice cube trays and freeze them. Then, when it's time to take your next dose of nystatin, you can pop a "nystatin-sicle" into your mouth. As it melts, it can provide soothing coolness and comfort to your tissues.

Food Aversions

During this period of time when you may be experiencing nausea or taste changes, you may find that some foods are particularly aversive. This conditioned response is not unusual when an unpleasant experience is strongly associated with a particular food or taste. For example, if you ate a tuna sandwich which caused food poisoning (hours of abdominal pain, nausea, and vomiting), you might not want to eat tuna salad again for a long time. This is an example of food aversion caused by an association with an unpleasant experience. It is not uncommon for people getting cancer treatments that cause nausea or other digestion problems to develop a food aversion to something they have ingested prior to that distress.

One way to avoid food aversions is to prevent the nausea from developing, or relieve it as soon as possible. Take the medications that have been prescribed, at the dose and times recommended. Another way to avoid developing food aversions is to eat a variety of different foods and flavors, especially when you are feeling nauseated. Those foods should be bland, easily digested, and leave no lingering taste or smell. That way, you do not associate one particular food or flavor with the unpleasant feeling.

Sometimes in an attempt to stimulate your appetite when you are feeling bad, a family member will prepare your "favorite" food after chemotherapy or radiation treatments. They may be surprised and disappointed that after a while you can no longer stand the sight or smell of that "favorite" food.

Poor Appetite—Anorexia

Anorexia is the medical term for loss of appetite. A person with anorexia does not feel like eating, and it is a problem for many people who are getting cancer treatments. Even though they know they need to maintain good nutrition at this time, it's hard to have an appetite if they are experiencing nausea, taste changes, constipation, fatigue, or pain. Relieving these symptoms can help improve your appetite.

Feeling full. Your digestive tract may slow down so that your food takes a longer time to move through. When you feel that food is "sitting in your stomach," you may have a feeling of fullness, and eating anything else may be difficult. With or without nausea or the feeling of fullness, your appetite may wane while you are getting treatment. A large plate of food (even something you might like) can make you feel overwhelmed or discouraged. One way of coping with this feeling is to eat five or six small meals spaced throughout the day.

Fatigue. If you are having problems with fatigue, just making a meal can be so exhausting that you lose the desire to eat. Some people cope with that problem by freezing single portions of homemade meals or buying frozen dinners. On days when you do not have the energy to cook, you can heat up a frozen meal with minimal effort.

Taste changes. If food seems tasteless, it is not as appetizing. Try eating foods which have stronger flavors—spicy, sweet, or sour—so that they are more interesting. Stimulate your appetite with foods prepared and served attractively, perhaps shared with a friend.

Your doctor may prescribe medicine to stimulate your appetite or speed up the movement of food through the digestive system to help relieve the feeling of nausea or fullness. Another resource is the dietitian, who may offer other suggestions to help maintain good nutrition until your appetite returns to normal. Chapter 7 ("Maintaining Good Nutrition") has more suggestions about how to spark your appetite during this time.

Diarrhea

When you have diarrhea, food moves through your large intestines so quickly that the water is not able to be absorbed normally. Therefore, your bowel movements are more liquid and more frequent. This problem can be very distressing and disruptive to your normal routine and can cause severe fluid loss and imbalances in the salts and minerals your body needs. There are a number of different reasons that people getting chemotherapy and radiation therapy can develop diarrhea.

1. Effects of cancer treatments. Chemotherapy and radiation therapy to the abdomen damages the cells in the intestinal tract that are dividing frequently. When that happens, the body responds by trying to remove the damaged tissue as quickly as possible. The rhythmic movement of your intestines (peristalsis) speeds up, and anything in the intestines moves out rapidly in the form of liquid stools. Diarrhea will abate when the intestinal lining heals.

2. Effects of medications. Diarrhea may also be caused by medications given to prevent nausea. Metoclopramide (Reglan) increases the movement of food and fluid through the digestive tract. This relieves the feeling of fullness from food sitting in the pit of your stomach. One problem with this increased movement is that it sometimes causes loose stools.

3. Effects of infection. Diarrhea can also be caused by infection. Chemotherapy and radiation therapy suppress your immune system, and you have fewer white blood cells to fight infection. As a result, bacteria that normally live within your digestive system can cause infections when your defenses are temporarily weakened by the treatments.

What to Do When You Have Diarrhea

If you are having frequent loose stools, let your doctor or nurse know right away. Keep track of the frequency and approximate amount of your stools. You may be asked to collect a small amount of stool for the lab so that it can be tested for infection. If the cause of diarrhea is not infectious, your doctor may prescribe an antidiarrhea medicine to slow down your bowel. If an antinausea medicine is causing the problem, your doctor may recommend that you decrease the dose or frequency, or you may be switched to another antinausea medicine.

When you have diarrhea, you may lose so much fluid that you can become dehydrated. Along with the fluid, you lose important minerals (especially potassium). If severe diarrhea goes untreated, you may experience other signs of dehydration such as feeling dizzy or weak. Your kidneys will make less urine in an attempt to hold onto fluid and therefore can't remove waste products adequately.

For all of these reasons it is important to keep drinking lots of fluid and replacing lost minerals. Try slowly sipping small amounts of fluids such as fruit juices and nectars, soups, or Gatorade (or another sport drink formulated to replace lost electrolytes). Since drinking very cold fluids can irritate your intestines and cause more discomfort, try drinking moderately cool or lukewarm fluids. If you feel like drinking sodas such as ginger ale, it's best to let the "fizz" out first so that you won't feel bloated. (The carbonation in the soda can also irritate your throat as it goes down.)

If you are at home, weigh yourself and keep a record of the amounts and types of fluids you are drinking so that your doctor will have information to help decide if you are becoming dehydrated.

Antidiarrhea Medications

Diarrhea can be your body's way of getting rid of the organism causing the infection or toxic products produced by the organism. Just as it is important to remove a splinter from your finger so that it can heal, moving the infected stool out quickly is the best way of promoting healing of the intestines. If you have an infection, stopping the diarrhea allows the infection to remain longer in your intestines and cause more damage. That is why it is important to notify your doctor or nurse if you are having this problem. He or she may send a stool sample to the lab to determine if you have the kind of diarrhea caused by infection.

If the stool sample shows that you have an infection, you will first be given an antibiotic to start eliminating the infection, *before* you are given any medication to slow down the diarrhea. If you do not have an infection, you can use antidiarrhea medicines. Lomotil or Imodium will slow down the rhythmic movement of your intestine and allow liquid to be absorbed from the stool, producing firmer bowel movements.

Metamucil or Citrucel can be helpful in controlling loose stools. They contain an indigestible fiber that helps add bulk which forms a firmer stool. Be sure not to drink extra fluid for an hour or so after taking these products or your stools will continue to be liquid.

Constipation

Constipation is a decrease in the usual frequency of bowel movements. When you are constipated, the stool stays in your intestines longer, and so it may become very dry and hard. There are a number of reasons you could become constipated during this time. Anything that slows the movement of your intestines will cause constipation, and some chemotherapy drugs such as Vincristine also cause your intestines to slow down. You can become constipated if you are taking pain medicines frequently, because they too will slow the digestive tract. If you are less active than usual, the normal rhythm of your intestines is slowed. If you are not eating or drinking as much as you usually do because of nausea, fatigue, or a poor appetite, you can become dehydrated, leading to constipation.

What to Do to Prevent Constipation

1. Increase Fluids. Just increasing the amount of fluids you drink will help your bowel movements become softer. Warm, non-caffeinated liquids such as herbal teas, fruit juices, or prune juice are helpful to keep your intestines moving and prevent constipation.

2. Eat High-Fiber Food. Foods such as raw vegetables and beans will increase the bulk in your stools and stimulate the intestines to move. But if you increase the fiber in your diet, be sure to increase the fluid you drink. If you increase the bulk without increasing the fluid, you will become more constipated then before. See Chapter 7 ("Maintaining Good Nutrition") for more information about food choices for a high-fiber diet.

3. Increase Activity. There are a number of reasons why you may be less active. Your usual routines might be changed drastically because of the necessity of keeping appointments at the clinic, hospital, lab, or diagnostic tests. Besides, you may just feel a lot more fatigued than usual during this time. Pain medications or antinausea medications may also make you sleepy and less active. Or, you may not have energy because you are not eating or sleeping as well. But even if you are not up to your usual exercise program, some activity may help relieve constipation. Just taking a short walk each day in the fresh air will make a difference.

4. Laxatives, Stool Softeners, and Enemas. Although many medications are available to treat constipation, check with your doctor before taking any to make sure that you are using the right one for you.

Stool softeners work by combining or mixing with the stool to make it more oily or more liquid. Colace, ducosate sodium, or DSS are examples of stool softeners. Oil-based suppositories such as Glycerine work in much the same way.

Laxatives stimulate the intestines to move the stool along at a faster rate and thus prevent the stool from getting too hard or dry. Drugs such as Castor oil, Cascara, or Ducolax increase the movement in the intestines by irritation. The intestines move faster in an attempt to remove the irritating substance out of the body sooner.

Bulk-forming laxatives such as Metamucil or Citrucel contain indigestible products such as bran or methyl cellulose, which increase the volume of the stool in your intestines. When your stool has more bulk, the feeling of fullness in your rectum stimulates the urge to have a bowel movement. Fruits or vegetables work the same way because the indigestible portions of those foods contribute to the bulk of your stool.

Milk of Magnesia contain nonabsorbable salts, which help retain fluid in your stool. With the increase in fluid, the stool is bulkier and thus stimulates the urge to have a bowel movement.

Enemas work to stimulate your lower intestine by irritation or by increasing the volume of the colon contents. That stimulates the colon to contract. Be sure to check with your doctor before using any medication rectally. During the times when your white blood cell count or platelet count are low, you could risk infection or trauma by using an enema or suppository. Prolonged use of laxatives or enemas may also inhibit your body's natural ability to have a normal bowel movement.

There are many products that are effective in relieving digestion problems. Some of these products are available now without a prescription. You probably have a medicine cabinet full of remedies with everything from antacids to suppositories. But during the time you are getting chemotherapy or radiation therapy. Talk with your doctor or nurse to be sure what you are taking will be safe and effective.

7

Maintaining Good Nutrition

by Barbara Yost, R.D.

Eating a balanced diet is an important part of good health. During your treatment, eating well is especially important. A balanced diet provides the proteins, fats, carbohydrates, vitamins, and minerals to give you energy, repair normal tissue, and fight infection. Eating well supports your body and helps normal cells recover quickly.

But food provides more than just the fuel for your daily activities. Eating special foods can also be a way you nurture yourself. And sharing meals is a way of socializing with others. People eat out in restaurants to celebrate or relax. Preparing food for others is one way that people show their love and concern.

When your ability to eat normally is changed, even temporarily, it can affect more than your nutrition. It can affect your sense of self and your ability to enjoy the pleasurable sensations and activities that occur around the experience of eating.

How Does Chemotherapy and Radiation Therapy Affect the Digestive System?

From your mouth to your large intestine, your digestive system is lined with rapidly dividing cells that are vulnerable to the effects of chemotherapy or radiation therapy. These therapies can cause a change in appetite, alter your sense of taste, and cause nausea, diarrhea, or constipation. These side effects can make it hard to eat a balanced diet.

The severity of the side effects of chemotherapy and radiation therapy depend on the particular medicines, dosages, and individual sensitivities. You may also be taking other medications that can cause digestive problems. For instance, pain medicines can cause constipation, and some antinausea medicines can cause diarrhea or constipation.

Certain side effects are more likely at certain times. Nausea or fatigue may be problems for the first day or so after chemotherapy. Diarrhea may be a problem a week or so later. Radiation therapy may cause digestion problems that develop more slowly over the course of treatment. The explanations for these differences are covered in Chapter 5 ("Coping with Nausea") and 6 ("Coping with Other Digestion Problems").

Because your symptoms may change, your eating strategies may need to change as well. After several cycles of chemotherapy or several weeks of radiation therapy, you will have a much better idea of the difficulty (if any) you may have maintaining a healthy diet. This chapter will give you some idea of the problems that may arise and some suggestions to help you overcome them.

Cancer, Cancer Treatments, and Weight Loss

Cancer is often associated with a profound loss of weight. As cancer cells are rapidly growing and dividing, they use the vitamins, minerals, proteins, and calories that the rest of your body needs. They sometimes also release chemicals that speed up your body's use of these nutrients or suppress your appetite. Cancer cells can also interfere with your ability to chew, swallow, or digest your food normally. And your appetite can be poor due to taste changes, fatigue, or the stress of being ill.

Staying well nourished and maintaining your weight while you are receiving cancer-fighting treatments is particularly important to your recovery. Your doctor or nurse will weigh you at each visit and monitor your weight carefully as an indication of your ability to tolerate the chemotherapy or radiation therapy. Think of food as part of your healing—one feature of your recovery over which you have some control.

Your goal is to eat the amount and balance of nutrients required to support your exceptional needs over the course of your treatment. Start by following your personal food preferences, tastes, and routines. You know your likes and dislikes best and have a good idea of food you can and cannot tolerate. The more you normalize your eating and your activities around food, the better you'll feel and the more successful you'll be in meeting your goal.

Anticancer Diets

The challenge while getting chemotherapy and radiation therapy is to eat enough calories to maintain your weight and provide energy to fight infection and recover from the effects of your treatments. You've probably read about diets that protect you from cancer: high fiber, increased vitamins A, C, and E, more broccoli and sweet potatoes, less total fat. But when you are dealing with the problems of nausea, poor appetite, or feeling full quickly, some of the features of an anticancer diet are inappropriate. For example, foods higher in fat provide more calories for less volume than low-fat foods; or, when you are having diarrhea, you won't want to be eating broccoli.

Aim to keep a five- to ten-pound weight range around your usual weight. During the months of your treatments, your weight will fluctuate. There will be days when you won't have much of an appetite and will want to eat lightly. On other days, you'll eat normally. The few pounds that you lose at one point can be made up when you are feeling better. Follow the suggestions at the end of this chapter to boost the number of calories in your diet during the catch-up phase.

Stimulate Your Appetite

Even though your appetite may be poor, there are things that you can do to stimulate your desire for food:

Go to a market or delicatessen and search out foods that appeal to you. Look through cookbooks and magazines for ideas for tasty foods.

Eating out can stimulate your appetite. In a restaurant you have the opportunity to choose from an enticing variety of foods, and you don't have to do the shopping, preparation, or cleanup.

Vary the surroundings where you eat. Eat on the front porch or in the garden. Use a cloth napkin or table cloth for another change. Make mealtime a treat to all your senses. Listen to relaxing music, dim the lights, brighten the table with flowers. Remind yourself to stay calm and unhurried.

Give thought to how the foods look on the plate. A variety of colors, textures, aromas, and shapes makes a meal interesting. Add a garnish. Set a colorful place.

Eating with other people and sharing conversation can also be stimulating. Induce a good friend to come once a week with a prepared meal for the two of you to share. Read or watch TV or an old movie while you eat.

Light exercise can also increase your appetite. Walking in the fresh air before a meal may help you feel hungry and more energetic. If you can't get out of the house, light housekeeping or craft work can be stimulating to your appetite.

If you feel full too quickly, try eating frequent small meals. Become a "grazer"—eat a bite or two every few minutes. Keep snacks handy in different rooms of your house. You will eat more if food is readily available. Eat whenever you are hungry, at mealtimes and between meals, too.

You may find food more attractive if you serve yourself small portions. A huge pile of food on a plate or a giant glass of beverage can be a turn-off if you are not feeling particularly hungry.

Small Amount—Big Calories

When you can't eat as much as you usually do, increase the calories in the food that you do eat. Calories are a measure of the energy a food provides. Normally you need about twelve to fourteen calories per pound to maintain your weight. Healing from surgery or recovering from the effects of chemotherapy or radiation therapy takes extra energy, so you need even more calories.

One apple has about 80 calories; one slice of apple pie has about 400. If your appetite is poor and the pie appeals to you, eat the pie and get five times as many calories. Instead of drinking a plain glass of milk, make a milkshake with added ice cream. If a liquid diet is all you can tolerate, make the liquids high in calories. Use a blender to make sherbet shakes. Make your hot cereal or cocoa with milk or half-and-half instead of water. Add cream to your soups. Spread mayonnaise, peanut butter, or cream cheese on bread. Smother vegetables with cheese or cream sauces. Drink eggnog with your meals.

The chart at the end of this chapter contains sample menus for meals that are particularly high in calories and protein and they are nutritious as well.

Weight Gain

Some people gain weight during the months of cancer treatments. This can be caused by a number of things, but unusual weight gain should always be evaluated by your doctor.

Eating to Control Nausea

Some people experience mild nausea for a few days after chemotherapy. Avoiding an empty stomach sometimes helps overcome this discomfort. Women who are having morning sickness in early pregnancy also find this method of controlling nausea effective. If you are snacking continuously between meals, cut down on the amount of food you eat at regular mealtimes to keep your weight in the normal range. Also check with your doctor about alternative antinausea medications which may be more effective in controlling your nausea when you are having this problem.

Steroids

Steroids (prednisone, dexamethasone, etc.) are sometimes part of your chemotherapy treatment. A side effect of taking large doses of steroids over an extended period is that they change your metabolism (the rate at which you use calories). Some people may even develop a form of diabetes during the time they are taking high-dose steroids, so that they are required to eat a calorie-controlled diet or take insulin during this time. Steroids can stimulate your appetite, as well as cause you to retain fluids—both of which can cause weight gain.

Retaining Fluids

Another reason for your weight gain is that your body may be collecting fluid in an abnormal way. Cancer can cause fluid to accumulate in your lungs or abdomen. Pressure on a large blood vessel can cause swelling in your legs. If your weight is going up without any apparent reason, check with your doctor. Let him or her know how much weight you have gained since your last appointment. Also mention if your ankles are swollen, if you are feeling short of breath, or if your abdomen seems larger (or your waist band seems tighter) than usual.

Large volumes of fluid by IV over several days may cause a temporary weight gain. Your kidneys will usually filter out the excess fluid, but sometimes it takes a while to catch up. Your doctor may prescribe a diuretic to help your body eliminate the excess.

Changes in Taste

Tasting food is essential to our enjoyment of eating. Even as children, we have our favorite foods and flavors. When things taste different, it can be very disorienting. People on chemotherapy sometimes experience a temporary change in their sense of taste caused by medicines entering the saliva and altering the taste of food. Temporary changes in the mucous membranes of your mouth from chemotherapy or radiation therapy may have the same effect.

People report that sweets taste more or less sweet during this time. Red meat such as beef or lamb may taste bitter, and foods that are usually bitter may taste more so. A common complaint is that foods taste salty or metallic, or that the flavors of food are reduced.

Here are some suggestions that you can use to cope. If foods taste dull, try cooking the food in ways that heighten the flavor. Cook with wine, or use salad dressings or strong seasonings. Smooth, bland foods may taste chalky or pastelike. Garlic, onions, lemon, mint, and oregano are a few of the strong flavors that will help give food more taste and make it more appealing.

When your sense of taste is altered, use other senses to enhance meals. Keep appealing dishes covered until served, allowing the burst of aroma to tantalize you when the food is uncovered. Serve foods with distinctive textures. Crisp, smooth, crunchy, and chewy foods will stimulate your mouth. Eating some foods cold or frozen may increase their appeal.

Temporarily eliminate offending foods from your diet. If you have lost your desire to eat meat, substitute other high-protein foods such as eggs, cheese, milk, dried beans, tofu, or nuts. Replace salty foods with the salt-free variety. If something tastes too sweet, find a less sweet substitute. Return foods to your diet when they no longer taste "funny."

Bitterness is sometimes helped by eliminating metal pots or pans when cooking. Most food can be cooked in oven-proof glass or in plastic in the microwave. Marinate red meat in soy sauce, fruit juice, or wine before cooking to reduce bitterness. Chicken, turkey, and ham may still appeal to you when red meats do not.

If food tastes metallic, try sucking on lemon drops or a tart fruit candy before meals. Rinsing your mouth may also help decrease a metallic taste.

Any liquid nutritional supplements that you use to boost calories may taste better cold or over ice. You can get rid of any "vitamin" smell by drinking from a covered cup through a straw.

Be creative. Discover the flavors that you enjoy or that come through by experimentation. Find the foods that appeal to you and prepare them in ways that spark your appetite.

Nausea

Cancer therapy and nausea are so often associated that many people fear that nausea is an inevitable side effect of their treatment. This is not true. The chance of developing nausea depends on the specific area of your body that is receiving radiation, or the specific chemotherapy drugs you receive, the doses, and your particular reaction to them.

For those who are likely to develop nausea, prevention is essential. A number of the drugs that are prescribed for this purpose are often given even before chemotherapy or daily radiation therapy. Most people, including those getting large doses of the most nausea-inducing treatments, are usually comfortable and able to eat a fairly normal diet. In the hospital or clinic, nurses can give you nausea-preventing drugs (called antiemetics) at intervals so you don't experience the problem. The success of this approach can make it easy to forget that your comfort is dependent on taking the antiemetic. Some people feel so well while they are getting treatment that they wait until they feel nauseated before taking these drugs at home. The trick is to avoid the problem so you don't run the risk of getting dehydrated, developing food aversions, or experiencing "anticipatory" nausea. Read Chapter 5 ("Coping with Nausea") for descriptions of the drugs available to prevent nausea, an explanation of how they work, and suggestions for how to eat before and after your chemotherapy or radiation treatments.

Sometimes the feeling of nausea is mild, and people find that eating frequently settles the stomach. Morning nausea can be avoided by keeping crackers and juice by the bed so you can eat before getting up.

If you don't feel like eating solid food, it is especially important to drink fluids so you don't become dehydrated. Drink small amounts of cool, clear beverages frequently (every fifteen to thirty minutes) if possible.

When you know that putting anything in your stomach will make you vomit, wait. Don't try to eat or drink until the vomiting is under control. Vomiting will further deplete you of fluids and electrolytes. You may first have to take an antiemetic medicine by rectal suppository. If you continue to vomit and cannot keep anything down, call your doctor. You may need to take fluids and antiemetics by IV to prevent dehydration.

Once vomiting is under control, try small amounts of water (one sip every ten minutes, advancing to one to two tablespoons every twenty to thirty minutes). If you keep this down for an hour, increase clear liquids slowly and gradually work up to a small, bland meal (like chicken and rice soup and crackers). If you can tolerate this meal, advance towards a normal diet. When you are hungry and think that you can hold food down, choose bland, low-fat foods that are easily digested. Sometimes eating foods cold will prevent their odors from stimulating nausea.

Rest after eating and focus on deep, natural breathing. Here are some foods that are easily tolerated when you are feeling nauseated:

- Apple or grape juice
- Fruit nectars (peach, apricot, guava)
- Bottled fruit-and-water blends
- Cold melon
- Fruit smoothies
- Sherbet
- Popsicles
- Jell-O
- Applesauce
- Oatmeal or Cream of Wheat
- Canned fruits
- Angel food cake

Dry Mouth

Chemotherapy affects the mucous membranes in your mouth. Radiation treatments of the head, neck, or upper back can also affect those mucous membranes. These treatments can create a decrease in the amount of saliva you produce. Additional drugs, such as antiemetics or pain medicines, can also dry your mouth. Your mouth may feel so dry that it is hard to eat. A dry mouth can cause foods to taste strange and make chewing and swallowing uncomfortable.

Dry foods like bread or meat can make the problem worse. When you are not producing enough saliva to mix with your food and allow it to be swallowed easily, add gravy or sauces. Dip cookies in tea to make them moist. Cook vegetables until soft or even puree them.

If your mouth is dry, drink lots of fluids, both with and between meals. Keep a cup of juice, tea, or broth close by and sip often, swishing the liquid around before swallowing to moisten all surfaces of your mouth.

If your mouth is not sore, try tart or sweet beverages or foods (like lemonade) to stimulate your mouth's production of saliva. Chewing gum or sucking on hard candy or Popsicles also stimulates saliva.

If your lips are also dry, use lip salves to keep them moistened. Saliva also helps clean your teeth. Avoid dental problems by brushing your teeth and rinsing your mouth often, especially after eating.

Thick, sticky saliva may be a problem too. It can build up, especially during the night, and add to the problem of early morning nausea. Rinsing your mouth with warm water or a carbonated soda before eating will thin your saliva. Drinking hot beverages, such as tea with lemon, or sucking on hard candy will stimulate saliva and loosen thick mucus.

Try these foods when your mouth is dry or if you have thick, sticky saliva:

- Thin hot cereal
- Warm lemonade
- Melon
- Diluted fruit juice
- Popsicles or fruit ices
- Thin, broth-based soups (chicken and rice, beef noodle)
- Cooked fish or chicken in broth
- Blended vegetables or fruit diluted to a thin consistency

Sore Mouth and Throat

Your mouth and throat may feel sore and sensitive for a period of time during your chemotherapy or radiation therapy treatments. Chapter 6 ("Coping with Other Digestion Problems") discusses this problem and what to do to prevent and treat the soreness and infections if they occur.

When your mouth is sore, chewing and swallowing can be painful. Some foods are especially irritating and should be avoided. Other foods are soothing. Try these suggestions if your mouth is sore:

Eat cool, smooth foods to reduce discomfort. Stay away from spicy, hot, or salty foods or acidic foods like citrus fruits and juices.

Avoid rough, coarse, or dry foods like raw vegetables, granola, or hard toast. Let hot foods cool down before eating or drinking them.

Puree food in a blender or food processor. Baby food is also bland, smooth, and easy to tolerate.

Use a straw to drink liquids. This will deliver fluid to the back of your throat and avoid sore areas.

Nutritional supplements are a good source of high-calorie, high-protein, nonacid liquid. You can buy products like Ensure Plus or Sustacal in a drugstore or mix your own by adding milk to Instant Breakfast. Look for brands that have more than 300 calories per cup of prepared liquid. A chart at the end of this chapter compares some popular nutritional supplements.

Here are some other cool, soft, nonacid, nonspicy foods that you can try:

- Milkshakes, nectars, grape juice, Popsicles, Jell-O
- Canned or soft fruits (bananas, applesauce, melon)
- Cottage cheese, mashed potatoes, macaroni and cheese
- Scrambled eggs, cooked cereal
- Pureed vegetables and meats (like baby food)
- Custard, pudding, milk toast, ice cream

Diarrhea

Diarrhea causes the food and liquids you have eaten to pass through your bowel so quickly that fluid cannot be absorbed from your digestive system normally. When this happens, you lose more than just water—you lose salts and minerals essential to the functioning of other body systems. Too much fluid loss may result in severe dehydration and weakness.

Diarrhea can be caused by a number of conditions including infection, food sensitivities, and antibiotics or other medications. Medications that prevent nausea sometimes work by speeding up the movement of food through the digestive system, which can also cause diarrhea.

The cells in your intestinal tract are vulnerable to chemotherapy and to radiation therapy. Because these frequently dividing cells are not being replaced at the usual rate, you may start to have diarrhea about a week after treatment. You are also more likely to develop intestinal infections at this time.

Unrelieved diarrhea can be a serious problem. Call your doctor if it continues. She or he may want to test a sample of your diarrhea for infection or prescribe a medication to slow down your intestines. If you have become dehydrated, you may need to replace fluid and salts through an IV.

Sometimes your doctor will want you to rest your bowel by eating only clear liquids for a day or two. Make up for the loss of calories when you are eating normally again to stay within your target weight range.

When you are having diarrhea, you want to eat low-fiber, nonirritating foods. Here are some suggestions:

During this time avoid caffeine (coffee, strong tea, chocolate), as it may aggravate the diarrhea. Also avoid greasy, fatty, or fried foods, raw fruits and vegetables, strong spices, carbonated beverages, and milk products.

Try the BRAT diet: Bananas, Rice, Applesauce, and weak herbal Tea, all of which are easily digested and unlikely to stimulate more diarrhea. The foods suggested for soothing a sore mouth (with the exception of milk products) are also good choices when you have diarrhea.

Eat small, frequent meals and drink plenty of liquids at room temperature between meals to make up for lost fluids. You need lots of extra sodium and potassium to replace what you are losing to diarrhea. Canned soups are high in sodium and easily digested.

Bananas, apricot nectar, or mashed potatoes will supply potassium. Mix mashed potatoes with chicken broth to make a creamy, milk-free soup that provides fluid, sodium, and potassium. Also try these foods:

- Yogurt
- Smooth peanut butter
- White bread
- Noodles
- Tender meats
- Fish

Constipation

Constipation occurs when your intestines slow down and you have fewer bowel movements. Since the food lingers longer than usual in your bowel, more water than usual is absorbed, and your stool becomes hard and dry. People who are constipated feel uncomfortably full, which can reduce their appetite. Pain medications often cause constipation, and lack of activity makes it worse.

The key is to prevent constipation. Your doctor may prescribe a stool softener, which holds water in the digestive system. Other medications stimulate the bowel, so that the stool will pass more quickly through it.

If you're constipated, drink plenty of liquids between meals, get daily exercise if possible, and eat a high-fiber diet. Also try these foods to prevent constipation:

- Whole grains—whole wheat, bran flakes, wheat bran
- Raw fruits and vegetables
- Dried fruits, prunes, prune juice

Fatigue

You may find that there are periods of time when you feel extremely fatigued. If you are the cook in your family, you will have to plan ahead so that you can get the rest as well as the nutrition you need when you are feeling tired. The following are some ways you can simplify things around mealtime.

Prepare meals in advance and freeze meal-size portions that can be easily thawed and warmed up in the microwave or oven.

Casseroles are especially good, because they combine protein and carbohydrates in one dish. Store-bought frozen entrees, pizza, or take-out food can also be an easy dinner for your family when you are too tired to cook.

Ask a friend or family member to cook a dinner for you and your family when you are feeling tired. Help them by preparing a list of foods and spices that you would enjoy or would prefer to avoid.

Keep foods on hand that need very little preparation. Yogurt, canned fruit, canned soups, crackers, custard, eggs, and cheese are easy to prepare and are still nutritious. Keep snack food nearby (on the TV or on your night stand) so that you can reach for it easily without having to get up.

Minimize cleanup whenever possible. Use paper plates and cups more frequently and use cooking containers that can go from the freezer to the oven to the table so that there is less to wash. Ask others to help. Even young children can clear the table or stack the dishes in the sink.

Chapter 9 ("Coping with Fatigue") has more information and suggestions about how to cope with the problems of fatigue.

About the Author

Barbara J. Yost is a Registered Dietitian and Certified Nutrition Support Dietitian. She graduated in Dietetics from the University of California, Berkeley, and completed a Masters Degree at Tufts University. Barbara has a wide range of experience in the nutrition field, having taught nurses and worked in an outpatient clinic with all ages. Currently, she works at Alta Bates Medical Center in Berkeley, California, with cancer patients and patients in intensive care.

Other Resources

Here are several additional sources of information to help you plan, shop, and cook food during this time when your dietary needs and problems are changing.

Aker, S., and P. Lenssen. 1988. *A Guide to Good Nutrition During and After Chemotherapy*. 3rd Edition. This describes ways to eat while you are experiencing different side effects of chemotherapy. Write to Clinical Nutrition Program, Division of Clinical Research, Fred Hutchinson Cancer Research Center, 1124 Columbia Street, Seattle, Wash. 98104.

American Cancer Society. *Eating Smart*. 1987. This covers dietary recommendations that minimize cancer risk for the general population, and is useful after chemotherapy. Free. Call (800) 227-2345.

Haller, James. 1994. *What to Eat When You Don't Feel Like Eating*. The Robert Pope Foundation. Call (902) 684-9129.

Nixon, Daniel W., M.D. 1996. *The Cancer Recovery Eating Plan: The Right Foods to Help Fuel Your Recovery*. New York: Random House.

Ross Laboratories. 1989. *Nutrition: An Ally In Cancer Therapy*. This tells you different ways to use nutritional supplements. Write to Ross Laboratories, Columbus, Ohio 43216.

Spiller, Gene, and Bonnie Bruce. 1997. *Cancer Survivors' Nutrition and Health Guide: Eating Well and Getting Better During and After Cancer Treatments*. Rocklin, Calif.: Prima Publications.

U.S. Department of Health and Human Services, National Cancer Institute. 1994. *Eating Hints for Cancer Patients*. Free. Call (800) 422-6237.

Sample Menus

Regular, Healthy Menu	Bland, Soft Menu (For sore mouth, delicate digestion)	High-Calorie, High-Protein Menu (For weight gain)	Light Diet Menu Therapy (Use for chemotherapy or nausea days)
Breakfast Bran flakes Non-fat milk Cantaloupe Whole wheat toast Butter, Jam	**Breakfast** Cream of Wheat Poached egg Instant Breakfast Apricot nectar	**Breakfast** Eggs, sausage Pancakes Syrup, Butter Orange juice Instant Breakfast	**Breakfast** Herbal tea Cold melon Cream of Wheat Sugar
Lunch Black bean soup Turkey sandwich on whole wheat bread Raw carrots and cherry tomatoes Buttermilk	**Lunch** Cream of potato soup Cottage cheese and canned fruit Milkshake	**Lunch** Cheeseburger French fries Milkshake Apple pie	**Lunch** Cottage cheese and fresh fruit Herbal tea Sugar Crackers Popsicle
Dinner Spaghetti with meat sauce Tossed salad with broccoli, Oil and vinegar, Garlic bread, Sherbet	**Dinner** Macaroni and cheese Cooked carrots Tapioca pudding Apple juice	**Dinner** Fried chicken Coleslaw Potato salad Biscuit and butter Apricot nectar	**Dinner** Apple juice Chicken and rice soup Jell-O
Snack Ideas Fresh fruit Dried fruit Raw vegetables Yogurt Bread Fruit juice	**Snack Ideas** Nectar Pudding Pound cake Bananas Mild cheese Canned fruit Ice cream	**Snack Ideas** Ice cream, Cake, Cookies, Milk, Fresh fruit salad with sour cream and brown sugar Candy Nutritional supplements	**Snack Ideas** Nonacid juices Nectars Soups Frozen yogurt
	You may need to divide food into 6 or more small meals to be comfortable	*Don't fill up on fruits and vegetables*	*Make up for any weight lost as soon as you feel better.*

*Omit meat if vegetarian; use soy milk or supplements if lactose intolerant

Liquid Nutritional Supplements Comparison Table

Sample Items	Approximate		Added Vitamins and Minerals	Lactose?
	Calories/cup	Protein/cup		
Whole milk	160	8 grams	A, D	Yes
"Double" strength milk	250	16 grams	A, D	Yes
Instant Breakfast–type powders	280	15 grams	Yes	Yes
Ensure, Isocal, Resource, Attain, Replete	250	9 grams	Yes	No
Ensure Plus, Resource Plus, Nutren 1.5, Sustacal HC	350	13 grams	Yes	No
McDonald's milkshake	350	9 grams	No	Yes
Haagen Daz, Ben and Jerry's ice creams	500	4 grams	No	Yes

Major Nutrients, Their Sources, and Functions

Nutrient and Safe/ Recommended Intake	Important Sources	Functions in the Human Body
PROTEIN 1/2 gram/pound	Meat, fish, poultry, eggs, dairy, nuts, legumes, seeds	Builds and repairs body tissues; make enzymes and antibodies
FAT less than 30% of calories	Butter, cream, oil, bacon, margarine, nuts, mayonnaise	Concentrated calories for energy; supplies essential fatty acids, carries soluble vitamins A, D, E, K
VITAMIN A RDA: 5000 IU	Liver, egg yolk, milk. Beta carotene: apricots, cantaloupe, mangos, dark green and deep yellow vegetables	Promotes smooth skin, healthy mucous membranes; essential for growth; protects against night blindness; antioxidant
VITAMIN D RDA: 400 IU	Vitamin D fortified milk, brewer's yeast, fish liver oil, synthesized by action of sunlight on skin	Absorbs dietary calcium and phosphorus; for strong bones and teeth
VITAMIN E RDA: 18 IU	Wheat germ oil, vegetable oil, leafy green vegetables, whole grain cereals, liver	Helps prevent destruction of vitamin A and C; helps prevent some infantile anemias; antioxidant
THIAMINE (B1) RDA: 1.5 MG	Brewer's yeast, wheat germ, pork, beef, liver, whole grain products, legumes, enriched flour	To use carbohydrates for energy
RIBOFLAVIN (B2) RDA: 1.7 MG	Brewer's yeast, liver, milk, cheese, leafy green vegetables, enriched flour	For healthy skin, eyes, mucous membranes; helps body use protein, carbohydrates and fat for energy

Nutrient and Safe/ Recommended Intake	Important Sources	Functions in the Human Body
NIACIN RDA: 20 MG	Brewer's yeast, peanut butter, meat, whole grain and enriched breads and cereals	For healthy skin and nerves; helps cells use oxygen to release energy
PYRIDOXINE (B6) RDA: 2.0 MG	Meat, liver, whole grain cereals and breads, bananas, spinach, fish	For protein and fat metabolism; for red blood cell formation
FOLIC ACID RDA: 400 MCG	Broccoli and leafy green vegetables, liver, asparagus, lettuce, legumes	Aids in development of red blood cells
VITAMIN C RDA: 60 MG	Citrus fruit, berries, tomatoes, potatoes, chilis, peppers, leafy green vegetables, broccoli, lettuce	For healthy skin, gums, teeth, blood vessels; for wound healing and bone growth; helps use iron; helps resist infection
ZINC RDA: 15 MG	Liver, shellfish, brewer's yeast, wheat germ, eggs, whole grains	For wound healing; involved in normal growth and development
IRON RDA: 15 MG	Liver, red meat, shellfish, leafy green vegetables, whole grain and enriched cereal products, legumes	In red blood cells, iron carries oxygen to cells; for good immune and nerve functioning
CALCIUM RDA: 1000 MG	Milk, cheese, yogurt, leafy green vegetables, shellfish, sardines	For strong bones and teeth; aids in normal functioning of muscles, nerves, enzymes; aids in blood clotting

8

Coping with Hair Loss and Skin Changes

Most of the temporary changes caused by the side effects of chemotherapy and radiation therapy happen inside your body. They aren't obvious to others. You cannot see a low white blood cell count or changes in appetite or digestion. But changes in your hair and skin happen on the outside of your body and are visible to others. Many people find that cancer treatments' effects on their hair are especially difficult. The way you wear your hair is one of the ways you express your identity and individual style. Dealing with hair loss or thinning can be a hard, even traumatic adjustment. Even though these changes may be temporary, you may still have to deal with them during the months of your treatments.

Not all chemotherapy medicines or radiation treatments cause hair loss. Your doctor or nurse will tell you about the changes in hair and skin that you can anticipate from your treatments. As with the other potential side effects of treatment, if you know what to expect, you will be better prepared to cope with the problems. This chapter will explain how chemotherapy and radiation therapy can affect your hair and skin, and what you can do to cope with the changes during this time.

How Does Chemotherapy Affect Hair?

Chemotherapy works by damaging cells that are rapidly dividing. As a result, cancer cells, which divide with greater frequency, are extremely vulnerable to the effects of chemotherapy. But the normal cells in your body, some of which are also dividing frequently, can be temporarily damaged. Since chemotherapy travels via your bloodstream to every cell in your body, all of your hair and skin can be temporarily affected.

Hair grows from follicles, which contain special cells that divide frequently to make your hair grow. Since at any one time about 90 percent of your hair follicles are in the active growth phase, they are especially susceptible to the effects of chemotherapy. Hair loss occurs when chemotherapy damages dividing follicle cells, producing weak, brittle hair that may break off at the scalp or fall out at the root itself. And it's not only the hair on your head that may be affected by chemotherapy. Some people notice that their eyebrow hair becomes thinner and they have fewer eyelashes or pubic hairs. But in general, since the hair on the rest of your body is not growing as rapidly as the hair on your head, you may not notice significant hair loss from other areas due to chemotherapy.

What Can I Expect with Chemotherapy?

Whether or not you lose your hair depends on the type and dosage of the chemotherapy drugs you receive. Some drugs may not affect your hair at all. Some may cause partial hair loss (hair thinning). And some chemotherapy drugs will cause complete hair loss. Your doctor or nurse will tell you what to expect from the specific drugs and dosages you are getting.

Although damage to the hair follicle is immediate, you won't see the result of that damage until a few weeks later. Your scalp may feel very sensitive, itchy, or tingly at first, and then you'll notice unusually large amounts of hair coming out on your brush or pillow, or more hair in the shower drain.

As more hair shafts break and less hair grows in because of the damage to the hair follicles, the remaining hair on your head will appear thinner. In some cases hair loss will show up in patches.

Just like the cells of your digestive system or bone marrow, damaged hair follicles recover quickly from the effects of chemotherapy. They start producing hair again right away. However, because the hair grows slowly, you probably won't notice hair growth before your next chemotherapy treatment, when the cycle is repeated. People who receive chemotherapy treatments every three or four weeks usually won't see hair growth begin to return until about a month or two after all chemotherapy treatments are completed.

How Does Radiation Therapy Affect Hair?

Radiation also damages cells that are dividing frequently, but unlike chemotherapy, the effects of radiation therapy do not travel throughout your body. Only the hair directly exposed is affected. Whether or not hair loss is temporary or permanent will depend on the amount of radiation to which your scalp is exposed. Radiation doses as low as 500 centigray (cGy) can cause temporary hair loss, and hair growth may be delayed for several months after treatment is completed. Radiation doses of 4500 cGy may delay hair growth for as much as a year, or it may cause permanent hair loss in the areas exposed. Your radiation oncologist will let you know whether or not to expect hair loss, if the hair loss will be temporary, and when you can expect the hair to return.

If the whole scalp is exposed to radiation, all the hair will be affected. If the radiation is directed to small areas of the scalp, hair loss may occur in patches, and the shielded areas of the scalp will not be affected. If the radiation goes through your body, it can also affect the hair or skin on the opposite side. This is called *exit radiation* and can also cause hair loss.

Regrowth of Hair

When your hair returns, it will feel at first like peach fuzz. Later you may notice other differences in texture. If your hair was curly before, the new hair may grow in straighter. Previously straight hair may grow in curly. Your hair may be finer or coarser than it was before, and your hair may grow in darker or lighter than your natural color. But if your hair grows back differently at first, over time it may return to its original color and texture.

How to Cope with Thinning Hair

Many cancer treatments cause your hair to become dry, brittle, and thinner than usual. When your hair is more fragile, you should be especially gentle in you hair care. Here are some suggestions:

- Wash and dry your hair gently—it's even more fragile when it's wet.

- Check with your barber or hairdresser for special products made to be used with "overtreated" or "damaged" hair.

- Avoid harsh chemicals like peroxide or permanents.

- Don't use a hot blow dryer or hot curlers. They'll make your hair even dryer and more likely to break.

- Many people find that shorter hair camouflages the problem of thinning. Longer hair is heavier, and the weight pulls it flatter on your head. Hair that is shorter tends to spring upwards and contributes to a fuller look.

- If your hair is long, you may want to cut it a little at a time. The change won't be so drastic, and you'll have a chance to adjust gradually to a different look.

- If your radiation therapy will cause hair loss in patches, you may want to grow some sections of your hair longer to cover those areas.

- Don't forget the importance of eating a well balanced diet to keep your hair healthy. Poor nutrition due to nausea or a diminished appetite may contribute to your hair looking dull and lifeless. Chapter 7 ("Maintaining Good Nutrition") contains suggestions about how to maintain a balanced diet while getting chemotherapy or radiation therapy.

Coping with Hair Loss

Even when people expect to lose their hair from chemotherapy or radiation therapy, it's still upsetting when it actually happens.

Since there is a delay of a few weeks from the beginning of treatments to when the hair starts to fall out, you will most likely not be in the hospital or clinic when it happens. So you will not have the support of nurses or other medical staff who are familiar with what is happening to you. It's distressing to see your hair clogging the drain or filling the brush. If your hair is long, it may be helpful to have it cut into a shorter style even before starting the treatment that will cause hair loss.

It may help to talk to someone who has faced this same problem. This is a good time to get involved in a cancer support group. Don't hesitate to check back in with the nurse at your oncologist's office or the radiation department for support or suggestions. Keep in mind, chemotherapy causes *temporary* hair loss. Your hair will regrow after your treatments are over. Radiation will cause hair loss only in the places that have been exposed to radiation and in many cases will regrow after treatments are completed.

About Wigs

If you plan to get a wig, it will be helpful to take some photographs of your hairline and your hair style from the front, side, and back. Also, snip little samples of your hair from the front and back as well. This will enable you to match the wig's color and style to your own hair.

Purchase your wig from a store which can provide experienced sales staff, privacy, and individual attention. If you are unsure about where to go, ask your nurse or the American Cancer Society for a referral. A member of your support group may recommend a particular store or salesperson who has been especially helpful.

In order to make your wig as natural looking and comfortable as possible, there are a number of things to consider when buying it.

Type of wig. Wigs can be made of different materials. A synthetic-fiber wig is less expensive, but tends to be stiff. It must be dry cleaned instead of shampooed and cannot be styled with a curling iron or permanent. Although a wig made from Asian or European hair is more expensive, it looks more natural and can be washed as well as styled. Asian hair will be coarser and straighter than European hair.

Wig construction. The way a wig is constructed affects its comfort and how natural it looks. If the wig has a mesh base, it must be dry cleaned and cannot take a perm. More expensive customized wigs have hair that is implanted into a skinlike base and are more comfortable.

Fit. It is very important that the wig fits you well. If you are constantly aware of it, if you are afraid to move in a natural way because it's uncomfortable, then you won't feel good wearing it. The wig isn't serving its purpose. Buying a wig while you still have some hair can be a problem because it may not fit as well after all your hair is gone. Be sure to have the wig refitted if necessary to assure comfort.

How you attach a wig can make a big difference. One way a wig can be attached to your head is with small pieces of a special kind of tape applied to your hairline and the base of the wig. Whatever way the wig is attached, it should feel secure. You should be able to move your head and bend over without worrying that the wig will slip.

Comfort. Your body generates heat, and when you perspire the air evaporates the moisture you've generated to cool you down. You might not normally notice the perspiration from your head, but it can be a problem when you wear a wig. The air isn't able to reach your scalp, and you may notice the perspiration making your scalp itch or feel hot. This can make your wig uncomfortable. To overcome the problem, try wrapping a thin cotton scarf around your head under the wig. Or, you can get a piece of stretch stockinet material that can be tied at one end to make a cap. This can then be worn under the wig, and it will help absorb perspiration as well as provide a cushion between your wig and your scalp.

Cost. The price of wigs can vary from sixty to several hundred dollars. The cost may be covered by insurance if the doctor writes you a prescription for a "wig prosthesis." (*Prosthesis* is the medical term for the replacement of a missing part by an artificial substitute.) Most physicians are aware of the wording required when petitioning the insurance company to reimburse you for the cost of your wig. Be sure to remind your doctor that the prescription wording must also indicate the medical necessity for the wig—for example: "Alopecia (hair loss) due to chemotherapy or radiation therapy." If your insurance can offset some of the cost of the wig, you may be able to afford a more comfortable or more natural-looking one that may be more expensive.

Alternatives to a Wig. Many women use scarves and head wraps as alternatives to wearing a wig. It is a way to add color, texture, and accents to your wardrobe. A basic cotton square folded into two uneven triangles and tied at the back of your neck can be both colorful and comfortable. You can add a contrasting color by twisting another scarf or cord and tying that around the first scarf. You can also experiment with side knots or adding a hat or beret over the scarf.

While at home or at night, you might try a soft terrycloth or cotton turban. It's an easy and comfortable alternative to a wig or head wrap. The American Cancer Society often provides turbans free of charge to people receiving chemotherapy or radiation therapy. Baseball caps have also proven popular with both men and women. They're colorful and can be worn either with or without a head wrap.

If you choose not to use any head covering, you need to be aware of the weather and the sun. Hair serves as an insulation to protect your body from losing heat. In cold weather you can become chilled easily, so you'll need a hat or scarf when outdoors. Your hair also protects your scalp from the ultraviolet rays of the sun, so you'll need a hat or sunscreen (at least SPF15) while you are in direct sunlight to avoid sunburns. The sun can cause a burn even in cool weather, or when the sky is overcast.

Skin and Nails

Dryness

Dry skin can be caused by a number of different factors—the effects of chemotherapy, antinausea medication, dehydration, or poor nutrition. Skin can also be dry and sensitive from the effects of radiation. Dry skin is not only uncomfortable and sometimes itchy, but it's also more likely to be damaged by normal activities. Here are some general suggestions to prevent and treat dry, itchy skin:

- Lubricate your skin after washing with a water-based moisturizer.

- Take warm rather than hot baths or showers, because hot water can actually dry skin.

- Use a moisturizing soap, which can save your skin from the drying effects of regular soap.

- Avoid alcohol-based products, because they will dry your skin.

- Avoid letting wool or other scratchy fabrics come in contact with your skin.

- Soft, loose cotton clothing is less irritating than tight-fitting clothing that may bind or cause more irritation to skin that is already dry.

- Use a skin lubricant such as Bag Balm to heal dry, cracked skin. This product is available without a prescription. It was originally used to heal the chapped, dry udders of cows. It is very effective for relieving severely dry and chapped skin. Ask the radiation oncologist to recommend other healing products for your skin.

Sunburn

Chemotherapy. Some chemotherapy drugs will make your skin more sensitive to the sun. This means that sun exposure that would ordinarily not affect you could cause a burn. If the chemotherapy drugs you receive cause increased sun sensitivity, take precautions. Use sunscreen with a protection level of at least SPF15. Be generous with sunscreen to areas likely to be exposed to the sun, such as your face, back of your neck, shoulders, ankles, etc. Use lip gloss with sunscreen to protect your lips. Wear a hat with a brim wide enough to protect your face and neck, as well as long sleeves and long pants to protect your arms and legs. Remember that even on hazy days the sun's rays can penetrate to cause a burn.

Radiation. Skin exposed to radiation may be sensitive, dry, irritated, or reddened. You need to protect those sensitive areas from the sun, which can cause further damage. Use sunscreen, soft cotton clothing, a broad-brimmed hat, an umbrella, or anything else that will protect your delicate skin.

Tanning

The color of your skin is the result of the amount of melanin it contains. Dark-skinned people have more melanin than light-skinned people. Your pituitary gland produces a melanin-stimulating hormone (MSH) that determines your complexion. When you are exposed to the sun, your pituitary is stimulated to produce more melanin, thus bringing about the normal tanning process.

Radiation therapy and some chemotherapy drugs such as 5-Fluorouracil (5-FU) stimulate your body to make more melanin than usual, and as a result your skin may become darker temporarily. Radiation can cause darkening of the treated skin only—the areas of your body not exposed to radiation will not be affected. Chemotherapy, on the other hand, travels through the bloodstream and goes to every part of your body. Some chemotherapy medicines, therefore, will cause a more generalized tanning effect.

When chemotherapy causes tanning, you may see darkening in the nailbeds (the skin under your nails), on the skin over joints, or in the mucous membranes of your mouth. If you are getting chemotherapy into the veins of your hands or arms, you may develop a darkening in the skin over your veins. It may seem that the patterns of the veins in your hands or arms are outlined in a color several shades darker than your normal skin tone. If you are getting chemotherapy into larger veins near your heart through an implanted port or central catheter, you won't see this darkening pattern. Sometimes the darkening effect is evenly distributed over your body, like a regular suntan. People with darker skin may be more likely to develop the darkening effect than people with lighter skin. Just remember that the skin reaction caused by some chemotherapy drugs is temporary. You may notice it beginning two to three weeks after the start of treatment, and it will start to fade away after your treatment is completed.

Flushing

Your skin may become temporarily flushed for a few days after receiving the chemotherapy drug Etoposide (VP-16). Most of the time the flushing will occur in a localized area, especially on your face or neck. The flushing is not painful, although the redness can be fairly bright. Unlike the tanning effect, which can last for a long time, the flushing will usually disappear a few days after your treatment.

Hand/Foot Syndrome

Some chemotherapy drugs such as 5-FU or Taxotere can cause temporary swelling or blistering of your hands and feet. The swelling can be painful and make it harder to do some simple things such as opening a bottle or buttoning your clothes. Your palms or soles may also become dry and chapped. If you notice your hands and feet beginning to swell or hurt, let your doctor or nurse know right away. Sometimes using Bag Balm on these areas can help them heal faster.

Radiation Dermatitis

Radiation passes through the surface of your body and can cause a temporary skin condition called *radiation dermatitis*. The skin exposed to radiation may become reddened, itchy, and uncomfortable. Later, the area may become very dry and flaky. The nurses and physicians will carefully check for any skin reactions. If there is a problem, they will prescribe medications and lotions to promote healing. Sometimes treatment may be delayed until irritated skin can recover. Whether or not you will experience this temporary skin problem will depend on a number of factors, including the following:

1. **The kind of radiation beam.** The higher-voltage therapies cause fewer skin problems because the radiation beam is more precisely focused. If several radiation beams are directed at the tumor from different angles and through different skin areas, each skin area is exposed to a smaller amount of radiation, and therefore receives less damage.

2. **The part of your body that is being radiated.** Areas of the body where there are skin folds, such as the groin or underarms, may develop irritation sooner because those areas tend to stay warm and moist.

3. **The dose of radiation and duration of the treatment.** The longer the treatments go on, the more likely there will be a skin reaction. Most people may not experience a reaction until they have had several weeks of daily treatments.

Radiation Recall

If you are receiving chemotherapy at the same time or shortly after getting radiation therapy, you may develop a skin condition called *radiation recall*. Radiation recall appears as a redness or dry peeling of skin that has been radiated. This may be caused by the effect of the chemotherapy interfering with the repair of radiation-damaged skin cells. If this happens, you should consult with your doctor or nurse in the radiation department for suggestions about how treat the problem. They may prescribe an ointment to promote healing. It is always wise to treat the affected skin gently by using a mild soap and avoiding irritating clothing, exposure to the sun, and extremes in heat (heating pad, hot-water bottle, hot showers) or cold (ice packs or exposure to cold wind).

Allergic Skin Reactions

At any time—not just during cancer treatments—you can have an allergic skin reaction to a particular medicine, food, or irritant. An allergic skin reaction may appear as raised, red, or itchy bumps on your skin. If this happens, you should check with your doctor or nurse as soon as possible. The itchiness of an allergic skin reaction can be quite irritating, and untreated may cause other skin problems or infections.

Sometimes it is obvious what caused the allergic reaction, and you can prevent further problems. If you get a skin reaction immediately after starting a new medication or eating a certain food, you can guess that it may be the source of the problem. Sometimes, however, it is difficult to determine what exactly is causing the problem. You can develop an allergic reaction to a medication or food that you may have tolerated well in the past. You can develop an allergic reaction after working in the yard or wearing clothes washed with a detergent you are not used to. Sometimes you'll never be able determine with certainty what has caused the problem. Be sure to report any allergic skin reaction to your doctor or nurse. You may need an antihistamine or steroid to stop the allergic reaction and bring relief. Or you may need to change medications to prevent this from happening again.

Nail Changes

Your nails grow from under the skin at the base of your cuticle. Chemotherapy's effect on these cells can cause your nails to become brittle and grow at a slower rate than usual or to become very soft, making them more likely to rip. After several weeks, when the part of your nail that was under your cuticle during chemotherapy grows out to where it is visible, you may see a white or dark band or ridge in the nail. As your nail continues to grow and the band or ridge moves closer to the tip of your finger, you may find that the nail breaks more easily, peels, or catches on your clothing.

To prevent your nails from tearing, you should clip them close to your fingertips. Protect your nails and don't put added stress on them that may cause them to break (don't use your nails to open things like soda cans). Some people find that tape or Band-Aids effectively prevent snagging while that fragile band or ridge grows out. Your nails are the best protection against pain or infection in the nailbeds, so try to let the ridges grow out naturally without peeling them off early and exposing the nailbed to damage.

You should not use artificial nails at this time. If moisture collects under the artificial nail, you can develop a fungal infection that is hard to treat. You should not use alcohol-based polish or polish remover, as these will only add to the problem of drying nails and cause them to break and peel. Only use polish remover that is lanolin-based.

Looking Good

Appearance and body image are important to nearly everyone. You need to have effective ways to cope with the temporary changes in your appearance caused by cancer treatments. A number of resources offer solid help so that you can look better and feel better about yourself. The American Cancer Society has put together a program called "Look Good . . . Feel Better." It's taught by specially trained cosmetologists who help people dealing with changes in their appearance due to chemotherapy and radiation therapy. These classes offer tips on how women can apply makeup, use scarves creatively, and camouflage skin changes. Ask your nurse or call the American Cancer Society to see if there is a class available near you.

The book *Beauty and Cancer*, by Diane Dan Noes and Peggy Melody, (L.S. Press, 1988), has many ideas for hair care, wigs, makeup, nutrition, and exercise. The authors also provide the names of beauty supplies, beauty consultants, and support agencies that specialize in hair care and beauty for your special needs during this time.

9

Coping with Fatigue

It is common to hear people complaining about feeling tired and worn out. The stress of living in a highly technical, constantly changing world contributes to most people's experience of fatigue. But for a person facing cancer and its treatments, fatigue can take on a new meaning. In fact, fatigue is probably the most common complaint reported during cancer treatments.

Fatigue is similar to pain in that it is invisible. You cannot get a lab test that measures the amount of fatigue you are feeling. Tiredness doesn't show up on an X ray or scan, and it's hard to describe to other people. Before you began cancer treatments, your fatigue was probably just an occasional inconvenience relieved with a good night's rest. You were able to push past your feelings of exhaustion and "carry on," despite feeling tired. People receiving chemotherapy and radiation therapy describe a different kind of tiredness. It may not be relieved by catching up on sleep. During this time you may not be able to push past the fatigue to work or play as much as you did in the past.

Why Does It Happen?

Even though fatigue is such a common side effect for people getting cancer treatments, it is not very well understood. Although many different factors (both physical and psychological) contribute to fatigue, there is no known single factor that causes it, and there is no known medication or treatment that will relieve it completely. But there are things you can do to conserve and restore your energy, as well as get through the times when your energy is low. You may find that your fatigue varies from day to day. There are times when you may feel profoundly tired, and other times when you feel like your energy has returned and you can do anything. After you get used to how your cancer treatments affect you, you may learn to predict your patterns of fatigue and energy. This will enable you to plan more activities for when you expect to have more energy.

Physical Causes of Fatigue

Cancer itself can cause fatigue. Even before a person is diagnosed with cancer, one of the first symptoms he or she may notice is generalized fatigue. Depending upon the type of cancer or its location, cancer can interfere with how well your body is functioning. If the cancer is in the bone marrow, your body will be unable to make enough red blood cells to carry oxygen to each cell. If the cancer is affecting other organs, your body may not be able to fully eliminate waste or absorb needed nutrients. Fatigue can also be caused by anything that interferes with your being able to breathe, such as a chronic cough, infection, or fluid collecting in the lungs. Anything that interrupts your body's normal functioning is likely to make you tired.

Cancer cells often are reproducing more rapidly than normal. This rapid reproduction requires a lot of energy. A fast-growing tumor uses up more of your nutrition and energy, and that can result in your feeling depleted and tired.

Pain is another cause of fatigue. Not all cancers are painful, but if you have pain related to the disease, the pain itself can be exhausting. Pain also interferes with your sleep. Many people are able to minimize the pain they feel during the day by using distraction, but trying to ignore pain also takes a lot of energy. Pain is often more noticeable at night and can prevent you from sleeping well. Even if you spend eight hours in bed at night, your sleep may not be as restful when you are in pain. Obviously if you don't sleep well, you won't have as much energy the next day.

Nutrition and Fatigue

All cells in your body need nutrients to function. Any upset in your digestive system, such as nausea and vomiting, diarrhea, or constipation, will also disturb your ability to eat well and rob you of energy. Fevers due to the cancer or from infections can also leave you feeling weak and tired. Any increase in body temperature not only makes cells work harder, but causes them to need more oxygen and nutrients to perform their jobs. Therefore, your body has to work harder when you have a fever, and that will make you feel more tired.

Cancer Treatments and Fatigue

Besides the physical reasons for fatigue, people with cancer often feel tired because of the treatments they receive.

Surgery

If you have had surgery to remove the cancer, it may take many weeks to regain your energy. If you had general anesthesia during the surgery, its effects may take some time to wear off. Your digestive system may need to recover from the surgery, so for a while you may not be eating normally.

Being in the hospital after surgery can also contribute to a sense of weariness. It is often difficult to sleep in the hospital because it is an unfamiliar environment. Your normal bedtime routines that help you relax into sleep are disrupted. You may also experience frequent interruptions of your sleep from hospital staff who come and go all night to check on you or to give you medications And the machines they use in the hospital make strange noises, beeps, and whistles.

Chemotherapy and Radiation Therapy

As cancer cells die, they create waste products. Your kidneys and liver have to work harder to eliminate these toxins, and that takes energy. Your body is also working harder to replace normal cells that have been affected by the chemotherapy, such as the lining of your digestive system and the blood-producing cells of the bone marrow.

People who are getting chemotherapy usually report that they feel more fatigued during the first day or two after the treatment. That is the time when they may be taking antinausea medications, which are often sedating. Chemotherapy patients also experience fatigue about a week to ten days after treatment, which is also the period of time when their white blood cell count is lowest—the *nadir*. As their immune system recovers, so does their energy.

Radiation therapy patients may not notice fatigue at first, but like other side effects of radiation, fatigue develops gradually over the weeks of treatment. Juggling your previous commitments to accommodate daily radiation treatments (along with driving, parking, and waiting in the radiation department) may also increase your stress. It will take several weeks after radiation treatments are completed for the fatigue to gradually fade and your energy to slowly return.

Biological Response Modifiers

These medications provide another form of therapy that can contribute to fatigue. Interferon or interleukin-2 help your own immune system combat the cancer or act like naturally occurring substances in your body which fight diseases. Unfortunately these treatments often cause a flulike syndrome which can result in fevers and fatigue.

Anemia

Red blood cells carry oxygen to every cell of your body. If you do not produce enough, you will tire easily and feel very weak and short of breath. This condition is called *anemia*. Cancer treatment can affect your bone marrow, causing a drop in the production of blood cells. If you become anemic because your bone marrow cannot produce enough blood cells, this decrease will diminish the number of available red blood cells needed to carry oxygen to the other cells of your body. Without enough oxygen, your cells are unable to perform their functions as they normally would. One of the effects of this process is weakness and a feeling of fatigue. Fortunately, anemia caused by cancer treatments is usually of short duration.

Anemia can also be caused by a lack of *erythropoietin*, which is a hormone that stimulates red blood cells to mature. If you are anemic your doctor may prescribe an injection of a synthetic form of this hormone that will increase the number of mature red blood cells.

Severe anemia may require a transfusion of red blood cells to supplement the oxygen-carrying capacity of your blood until your bone marrow recovers. The effects of the transfusion are quickly apparent—providing relief of the anemia and the fatigue. Your doctor will explain the risks and benefits of this treatment for anemia.

Other Side Effects of Treatment

Physical distress. Nausea and vomiting or even a low-level sense of queasiness can be taxing. For instance, if the side effects of cancer treatments interfere with your digestion, then you will not be able to process the food you need to give you energy. If the mucous membranes in your mouth and throat are sore, you may not be able to eat or drink adequately. If the effects of chemotherapy or radiation therapy cause diarrhea, you can lose a large amount of fluid and essential electrolytes. Untreated diarrhea results in dehydration and can leave you feeling very washed out.

Medications. Antinausea drugs such as prochlorperazine (Compazine) or lorazepam (Ativan) can be sedating. Dexamethasone (Decadron) is a steroid that is sometimes used along with other antinausea drugs to prevent nausea. But any steroid can make people feel "wired" and prevent them from being able to rest or sleep normally. During the day, this may not be a problem, but at night you may have trouble falling asleep.

No Time to Rest. Most likely, before your diagnosis your life did not revolve around going to the doctor or clinic. It takes considerable time and energy to go through all the necessary diagnostic tests and doctor's visits. This would be tiring even if you felt well! If you are also trying to keep up with other responsibilities such as work or caring for your family, this added stress may contribute significantly to your feeling of fatigue. When you are tired, you may feel that you don't have the energy to cope with all that is expected of you.

Stress and Sleep Disturbances

Feelings of worry and anxiety are a normal response to a serious illness. You may have concerns about many aspect of your life including your future, your family, and your job. Even though worry and anxiety are normal and expected responses to illness, these feelings can be exhausting. Worries often seem worse at night, and they can lead to difficulty sleeping. Your mind may race with questions. Why did this happen to you? Can it really be happening? After the initial shock of the diagnosis has passed, you may find yourself worrying about the future. How serious is the disease? What will the outcome be? What kinds of treatments are available? What are your options? If you have relatives or friends who have undergone previous cancer treatments or have heard stories about cancer therapies, you may ask yourself whether your experience will be similar, better, or worse.

You may have the additional concern of wondering how your family will manage. If you have children, just talking to them about your diagnosis may be painful or difficult. Economic concerns may be preying on your mind. If you provide support for your family, you may be concerned about how they will manage if you cannot work. Health insurance coverage or paying for medical care may be another financial worry for you. Your role in the family may be changing as well. While you are receiving treatment and dealing with your cancer, you may worry that you won't be able to function in your full capacity.

All of these very practical issues can create sleep disturbances. In addition, it is not uncommon to feel down or depressed. Many books written today emphasize the importance of being positive when facing cancer. But in light of the challenges people with cancer face, it is certainly not unusual to feel overwhelmed or out of control at times. Facing cancer may mean that you go through periods of feeling unhappy or depressed. These feelings will come and go, alternating with more positive times. But during the moments when you are down, you are also likely to feel more tired and fatigued. Chapter 12 ("Mind and Body") addresses these concerns as well as providing many suggestions you may find helpful in dealing with the stress of this period.

As you can see, fatigue associated with cancer and cancer treatments can be caused by many different things. Fortunately there are a number of things you can do to deal with the problem and feel better.

Managing Fatigue

Checking with Your Physician

It is important to talk to your physician about fatigue. You may be so focused on other symptoms and side effects that you forget to mention how tired you are feeling or whether you are having trouble sleeping at night. But depending upon the causes of your fatigue, there may be things your doctor can recommend to help you. The following sections contain some other ways you can help yourself prevent or relieve fatigue.

Improving Communication

When you recognize that fatigue is a common side effect of cancer and cancer-fighting treatments, you can begin to find ways to cope with it. First, you must communicate how you are feeling. If you enlist your friends and family members to help when you are tired, you will be able to conserve energy. Many people will be eager to lend a hand if only you ask.

Other people may not be aware of how you are feeling or understand the kind of fatigue you are experiencing. They may not understand the importance of limiting your activities or the ways you need to conserve energy. This is especially true if you are experiencing fatigue intermittently—some days you feel fine and other days you need more help, or more rest. Some people have difficulty asking for help, especially if they are used to being independent and responsible for others. It can also be uncomfortable if you feel your role at home or at work is changing because fatigue is limiting you. Often family members and friends are anxious to help but just don't know how. Be clear with others about exactly what you need from them. Then they can tell you clearly whether or not they can help. When you are specific about your needs, you are more likely to get the help you want without feeling overwhelmed by too much or neglected by too little.

Sometimes just talking to others who are also experiencing fatigue can be beneficial. It can be helpful to know you are not the only person struggling with this problem of weariness. Also, many people are happy to share with you what they have discovered to assist them in dealing with fatigue, stress, or sleep problems.

Lifting Your Spirits

You can think of the amount of energy you have as if it were money in a bank. There has to be a balance between what you deposit and what you withdraw. There are so many things that can diminish your energy and spirits. Physical and psychological stress, discomfort (pain, nausea, and so on), depression, frustration, worry, and boredom are some of them. Although you may not be able to completely eliminate these things from your life, see if you can limit the activities and/or people that sap your energy or add to your stress.

There are also many things that combat fatigue and help lift your spirits. An engaging conversation with a friend, meditation, or prayer can be restorative. Watching a movie, sitting quietly, or reading is restful. Mild exercise, such as a short walk in the fresh air, gets your muscles, lungs, and circulation moving, and that can make you feel invigorated as well as help you sleep better at night. Try to find time each day to do the things that lift your spirits and give you energy.

Keeping Track

Over a period of time, pay attention to when and where you feel tired. Although it will vary from day to day, you may find that there are predictable times when you feel more energetic than other times. Keep track of the pattern so you can plan your activities to accommodate the ebb and flow of your energy. For instance, many people have more energy in the morning after a night's sleep. You may feel restored after a brief nap, or after talking to a close friend. You may feel more tired after chemotherapy treatments, when your white blood cell count is low, or if you have an infection.

Pacing and Prioritizing

Pace yourself. Just as a long-distance runner doesn't go all-out in the beginning of the race, becoming too exhausted to finish, you have to pace yourself throughout the day. Try doing only one or two errands at a time, followed by a short rest. After your rest, perform one or two more tasks and rest again. Many of us want to finish everything on our lists before we take a break, believing that if we work this way, we will then be able to take a very long break after everything is finished. Unfortunately, by the time the long break comes around, you will be exhausted. If you start out feeling tired already, a marathon of errands will only lead to more fatigue. Listen to your body. Use your fatigue level as a gauge for taking breaks, and take the break when you are just starting to feel tired. Don't push yourself till you have zero energy. If you have trouble listening to your body, simply schedule regular periods for rest during the day and follow your schedule.

Prioritize the chores you need to do, ranking them by their importance and the amount of energy that each task will take. Then schedule them in the order that will be least tiring. For example, if you have more energy in the morning, plan to do something that will take more time and energy early in the day. Save the lighter tasks for the late afternoon when you may be more tired.

Making Choices

There will probably be times when you will not be able to do all the things that you want to accomplish. You just won't have the energy. Take another look at the "must do" list and decide what things you can reassign (to another family member), delay (to a day when you are not so fatigued), or just not do at all. You may have enough energy to either do the dishes or go to the park with the kids. You may prefer to spend your energy going out to lunch with your friends even if it means you do not get the car serviced.

Be efficient with your time and energy. Make a list before you go to the hardware store so you don't have to go back a second time for a forgotten item. You can use equipment or appliances to save time and energy when you are fatigued. A rolling cart can carry your groceries to the house. Try sitting down to water the lawn or to prepare food. Wait to hang the new shower curtain until your grandson can come and help you.

Sleeping Well

One way to help yourself sleep well at night is to avoid taking long naps during the day. If you are sleeping for long periods during the day, you may find yourself sleeping either fitfully or not at all at night. If you are not napping during the daytime, you will probably be tired enough to fall asleep when you retire. When you feel the need to rest during the day, instead of sleeping, try sitting quietly and relaxing by listening to soft music. Or just go into your room, close the door, and lie down for a few minutes.

Even if you don't nap for hours during the day, you still may find yourself struggling to fall asleep at night. Rather than tossing and turning in bed, get up. Try drinking a warm glass of milk or an herbal tea like chamomile. Reading a light book can be helpful. Or try some of the relaxation techniques described in Chapter 13 ("Relaxation and Stress Reduction"). It may take a little time to revert back to your usual sleep patterns, but with a little help, you can do it.

Going to the bathroom frequently at night can also interrupt your sleep. If this is a problem, it might help to limit how much you drink after dinner to avoid urinating in the middle of the night. If you are taking a diuretic (water pill), take it earlier in the day to avoid sleep disturbances.

If you're not sleeping well, look at your diet to make sure that you are not eating or drinking something that will keep you awake at night. Foods and drinks containing caffeine (chocolate, coffee, colas, and caffeinated teas) should be avoided in the evening. If you are thirsty at bedtime, it would be better to drink a warm noncaffeinated beverage.

Using Relaxation Techniques

If your fatigue is related to stress, anxiety, or an inability to sleep, relaxation and visualization techniques may be helpful. A very simple way to relax is to take ten minutes in the midst of a hectic day to sit in a quiet place by yourself without thinking about what needs to be done next. The old saying about stopping to smell the roses is appropriate when you feel stressed. Try to stay in the present, in the moment. Paying attention to the sensations of your environment (the color of the rose or the feel of the sun) takes your mind off of the activities or thoughts that are adding to your stress. Don't worry that you don't have the time or that there are things that need to be done. Take the time, and if worrisome thoughts intrude, take a deep breath and let them pass.

There are many types of relaxation techniques and breathing exercises that you may find helpful. A method called progressive muscle relaxation lets you systematically focus on and then relax groups of muscles. Another benefit of relaxation techniques is that they can often lead to a period of sleep. Full instructions for progressive muscle relaxation are covered in Chapter 13. You can find a script for relaxation and guided imagery in Chapter 14.

Using Medications

Your doctor can prescribe medications for sleep if you need them, and a number of over-the-counter medicines are available as well. If you are thinking of taking a medication for sleep, ask your doctor or nurse. They can tell you whether there will be a problem with interactions between the other drugs you are already taking and the sleep medicines.

If your sleep is disturbed by pain or other symptoms, be sure to take the medicines prescribed for treatment of these problems. Once the pain or nausea is under control, you will be better able to rest.

Eating Well

Nutritional problems may be contributing to your sense of tiredness. You may not be eating enough food to provide the materials your body needs to make energy. Are you nauseated or vomiting? Do you have a feeling of fullness even though you have eaten very little? Or is it that you do not have the energy to cook a nutritious meal? Sometimes people say they are just not hungry when they sit down to eat.

Since eating well is so important in relieving fatigue and helping your body recover from the effects of cancer treatments, it is important to carefully identify and eliminate as many of the obstacles to eating well as possible. If the problem is related to nausea or vomiting, be sure you are taking the antinausea medications as they were prescribed. Relieving nausea especially before you try to eat a meal is essential. Chapter 5 ("Coping with Nausea") provides many more ideas about how to prevent and relieve nausea associated with cancer treatments.

When cancer cells and normal cells die, they release substances into the body which can contribute to fatigue. Dehydration can also make you feel very fatigued. Even if you do not feel like eating solid food after radiation therapy or chemotherapy, drinking lots of fluids (juice, soda, broth, tea, popsicles) will help to flush out these waste products, prevent dehydration, and help you feel less weary.

Many people report that they feel full after eating a small amount of food. They find it overwhelming to look at a large plate of food when they sit down to eat. It can be helpful to prepare smaller portions of food at each meal, and in addition have three or four nutritious snacks between meals. You can add more nutrition to your diet with liquid supplements (Isocal or Ensure), which are high in calories, protein, vitamins, and other nutrients. If you have difficulty chewing or swallowing food, these supplements are easy to drink, and they come in different flavors for variety.

If your fatigue is due to anemia, try to eat foods containing iron and vitamin C. Vitamin C helps you to absorb the iron you ingest. You might also check with your nurse or doctor about taking a multivitamin pill to supplement your diet.

If you can tolerate milk products, another dietary sleep aid is a warm glass of milk before bed. Foods such as warm milk or crackers and cheese have substances (tryptophane and seratonin) which help the brain relax.

Many clinics and hospitals provide a nutritional consult at the beginning of treatment, and later to deal with eating problems as they arise. The registered dietitian can help you plan your meals to accommodate your food preferences, restrictions, energy resources, and time schedule.

Making Mealtimes Enjoyable

In our society, mealtimes are often the times we socialize with family or friends, so if you do not feel like eating, you miss both the nutrition and the company. Therefore, try to keep mealtimes as normal as possible. Join the family for meals even if you are not eating the same food they are. Returning to your usual ways of eating and socializing will help make the mealtime more enjoyable, and improve your appetite.

Another way to stimulate your appetite is to serve the food in an attractive way. Eat in the dining room with real dishes instead of in front of the television on paper plates. Invite a friend to share a meal. Eat out of doors or listen to your favorite music. Doing those things can make a meal feel more festive, and you may be pleasantly surprised by how much more you enjoy your food.

Getting Support

Depression, anxiety, and sleep disturbances are all conditions that can make the problem of fatigue worse. People who are depressed and anxious may not be eating or sleeping well. Since this is a period of time when you are facing extraordinary pressures and challenges, you may need the support of a counselor, psychologist, or member of the clergy who is experienced in helping people deal with illness. He or she can provide you with a safe place to explore your feelings, and help you find ways to manage your stress and concerns. An experienced counselor should be able to recognize the difference between sadness and clinical depression. If you feel that you might need help with depression, ask your oncologist to refer you to a psychiatrist for evaluation. You may have the kind of depression that could be helped by antidepressant medications. There are also medications that are very effective in relieving anxiety and sleep disturbances. See Chapter 12 ("Mind and Body") for more information about the emotional and psychological issues that you may be dealing with at this time.

In Summary

Fatigue is a frequent side effect of cancer and its treatments. More than one factor may be contributing to the problem, and often these factors are interrelated. Even if you try to eliminate as many as you can, there will still be times when you have to slow down and make changes in your daily activities because of fatigue. Those are the times when you have to be patient, rest, and eat well. Give yourself time to recover, and your energy will return as well. Even though there is no way of eliminating fatigue completely, there are things you can do to improve your energy, conserve your energy, and get through the low-energy periods.

10

Sexuality and Fertility

Any health problem can strongly affect your emotions. When you are coping with cancer and the stress of cancer-fighting treatments, you can feel overwhelmed. You may be worried or even angry about your diagnosis. You may feel pressured by the decisions you are being asked to make about your treatment or be fearful about your ability to survive. If you are recovering from recent surgery, you may still feel some pain and exhaustion. You may be adjusting to changes in your body from the illness or from surgery. If you have lost a part of your body (visible or not), you may still be grieving.

If you are in a relationship, your partner can be going through many of these same feelings of worry, depression, anger, and grief. These stresses can disrupt the balance of the relationship. Your need for contact, acceptance, and physical comfort may be even greater now, yet your partner may hold back. He or she may feel overwhelmed or hesitate to initiate physical contact for fear of harming you or adding to your stress.

If sexual contact was something you valued and enjoyed before your illness, your feelings probably haven't changed. But now you may have questions about how the illness or its treatments may affect your ability to be sexual. You may not feel comfortable asking your doctor or nurse about these concerns—questions about sex may seem unimportant or inappropriate in comparison to the life-and-death issues that they are dealing with. But information about how cancer or cancer treatments affect you sexually is important to your recovery. When is it safe to resume sexual intercourse? How will the medicine you are taking affect you sexually? Will you still be able to have an erection or experience orgasm?

Many myths about sex and cancer cause people much unnecessary anguish. Your mother may have complained that she was no longer interested in sex after her hysterectomy. Is that going to be true for you as well? You may worry that sexual activity may be harmful or painful after surgery, especially if the surgery involved the reproductive organs or breasts. You may worry that the cancer was caused by sexual activity. Some people fear that they can give cancer to their partner by intimate contact. These myths are not only untrue, but also damaging. If either you or your partner believe them, you risk losing the closeness and enjoyment of a sexual relationship.

One way of dispelling a myth is to ask your doctor or nurse about your concerns and get the facts clarified. If you do ask, you will learn that hormonal changes, menopausal symptoms, hysterectomy, or breast surgery do not necessarily mean the end of sexual enjoyment. Prostate or bowel surgery doesn't necessarily mean that a man can no longer have an erection or experience orgasm. Sex is not harmful to the person recovering from cancer, nor will it spread the disease.

The following sections will help you understand some of the basic facts regarding cancer and sexuality.

Sensation

All sensations, whether or not they are sexual, depend on the nerves carrying information to and from your brain via the spinal cord. Nerves to the sexual organs can be damaged from the pressure of a tumor on the nerves, the spinal cord, or the brain. These nerves can also be damaged as a result of the surgery done to remove the cancer. Fortunately, today's improved surgical techniques are less damaging to the organs and nerves that affect sexual functioning. Medications can also affect your nerves. Some chemotherapy medicines can cause numbness in the nerves and can affect your fingers and hands, as well as your legs and feet. The numbness can lessen your sense of touch. Other medicines that you may be taking to relieve pain or nausea can also diminish sexual responsiveness.

Hormonal Changes

A hormone is a chemical substance produced by one organ that is carried by the blood and affects other organs. For instance, insulin is a hormone produced by your pancreas. It is carried by the blood to other cells in your body and allows them to absorb or use sugar.

The sex hormones are responsible for the development of secondary sex characteristics and fertility in both men and women. These hormones are produced in the mature reproductive organs (ovaries in women; testes in men). Small amounts of both estrogen and testosterone are also produced in the adrenal glands, located near the kidneys. Although both sexes produce estrogen (the female sex hormone) and testosterone (the male sex hormone), men produce a great deal more testosterone, and women produce a great deal more estrogen.

At puberty, testosterone causes the male genitals to enlarge and the testes to produce sperm. It also stimulates the development of other characteristics, such as male distribution of body hair, voice changes, body build, and sex drive. Although the level of testosterone may slow down as a man ages, a man can continue to produce testosterone and sperm for his entire life.

In women, estrogen is responsible for the increase in size of the reproductive organs (uterus, cervix, vagina, ovaries), female distribution of body hair, body build, and the development of breasts. Since most of a woman's estrogen is produced in the ovaries, when these secretions slow down during menopause, the drop in the estrogen level causes a number of physical changes. Without estrogen, the vaginal lining is thinner, drier, and less elastic. The supply of blood to the vagina also decreases. The cervix (the bottom of the uterus) produces less mucous, and less lubrication is produced during sexual arousal.

The hormonal changes of menopause normally develop slowly over a number of years. But if the ovaries have been removed by surgery or stop functioning because of the effects of chemotherapy or radiation therapy, it can result in a sudden drop in a woman's estrogen level and cause changes in the vaginal lining and secretions. Characteristic hot flashes can be more frequent and severe than with normal menopause. Some women can take hormone pills which replace estrogen (as well as other hormones) to relieve many menopausal symptoms. But some kinds of cancer can also be stimulated to grow more rapidly in the presence of estrogen, so hormone replacement therapy (HRT) may not be possible.

Men can also be affected by hormonal changes. If surgery, medication, or chemotherapy reduces the production of testosterone, a man may experience some loss of sexual drive. Over time he will notice changes in hair distribution as well as changes in muscle and fat distribution. As with women, some cancers in men grow more rapidly in the presence of sex hormones, and in these cases doctors may prescribe antiandrogen hormones to turn off testosterone production. Some new, nonsteroid antiandrogen hormones are effective in lowering testosterone levels while having less detrimental effects on a man's sexual drive or ability to have an erection.

If a man loses his ability to maintain an erection because of surgery, reduced testosterone levels, or drugs, there are several options to consider. When the organic causes can't be corrected or reversed, some men choose to have a penile implant. One type of implant is a semirigid penile rod that keeps the penis partially erect at all times. A second option is a prosthesis that uses self-controlled inflatable rods. This type of implant inflates or deflates via manual manipulation of the penis. Instead of a prosthesis, some men prefer changing their sexual behavior to focus more on oral sex and manual touching for giving and receiving pleasure. This option has worked for many couples. Your doctor will be able to provide more information regarding these options.

Changes in Body Image

Your body image is the picture you have in your mind about your physical self. That picture helps form a sense of who you are. A positive body image allows you to feel whole, acceptable, and lovable. When that picture changes, there is necessarily a period of adjustment until you can adapt to the new sense of who you are.

People react very differently to physical changes. Some women experience a hysterectomy as a relief. They are rid of their menstrual periods and no longer have to worry about birth control. Other women may grieve for the loss of their uterus and menstrual periods because this loss signifies the end of the potential for having children and the disappearance of a function that is tied to their femininity and sexuality. Even if their uterus contained cancer cells and the surgery to remove it may have been life-saving, the hysterectomy can still be felt as a loss and a change in body image that takes time to integrate.

Body Image and Cancer

Just having cancer can be tremendously disturbing to your body image, especially if you've always felt strong and healthy. Surgery or other treatments that alter your body either temporarily or permanently can be even more traumatic, and when these changes are noticeable or disfiguring the natural process of grieving lasts longer. It can profoundly affect your self-esteem, confidence, and sexuality. If you dread looking at your scar after breast surgery or at your stoma (the opening on your abdomen where part of the bowel protrudes) after bowel surgery, you are likely to worry about how your partner will react, or how these changes will affect the way you share your body during intimate sexual contact.

Body Image and Cancer Therapies

The effects of chemotherapy and radiation therapy can greatly alter your body image as well. Hair loss is perhaps the greatest assault to your picture of yourself, but pallor and weight changes can also make you feel self-conscious about your body. A temporary intravenous line that is implanted in or emerges from your chest may feel foreign and obtrusive. Fatigue, nausea, or the sedating effects of pain and antinausea medication can prevent you from feeling sexual in your usual way. Your body may not feel like it belongs to you anymore, but to the doctors and nurses. It is no wonder that many people are reluctant to reestablish sexual contact while feeling this way.

Adjusting to Body Image Changes

The way you react to the physical changes caused by cancer and cancer therapies is personal. The amount of time it takes to adjust to these changes varies from person to person and from couple to couple. There is no right timetable, nor is there an ideal way that couples should deal with these problems. Some people are comfortable sharing the entire experience with their partner, having him or her present during doctors' visits, dressing changes, and any educational or supportive contact they have with other health care professionals. In that way, they learn together and are able to reinforce the information for each other. Partners can ask their own questions, and get clarification when needed. Other people want more independence, preferring to absorb the information at their own pace and share the information with their partner as they feel more comfortable over time.

For some people reconstructive surgery makes a big difference in how they feel about their bodies—all the physical adjustments seem easier. Other people feel that additional surgery would be traumatic, especially at a time when they may still be facing months of chemotherapy. Reconstruction may be something they'd consider after treatment is over, if at all. In any case, feeling whole and attractive and sexual is not dependent on reconstructive surgery.

Some people are more comfortable if they camouflage changes in their body when they are intimate. There are soft, fiber-filled "night bras" that can be worn under nightgowns to camouflage a missing breast. To cover a stoma and collection bag after a colostomy, some people wear a soft cotton cummerbund. Other couples feel closer to their partners if they can share themselves as freely as they did before their surgery and grow used to the changes together over time. Either choice is fine; it's a matter of doing what feels comfortable for you.

Dealing with Pain and Discomfort

Even when the doctor assures you that it's physically safe to resume sexual relations, you may not feel ready. You may need more time to heal, physically and emotionally. Or you may want to engage only in gentle sex play or sex that doesn't involve intercourse. Good communication is more important now than ever if you are to find a way to share sexual intimacy that is satisfying to both of you. Go slow. Let your partner know how you're feeling and what is comfortable for you. Your partner may be so fearful of harming you that he or she is reluctant to initiate sexual activity at all, and your encouragement and assurance is important.

If you take pain medication or a muscle relaxer, be sure to allow at least a half hour for it to work. Be aware that medications can also make you sleepy or limit your arousal. A warm bath or soothing massage is another way to feel more comfortable before sex.

You may find that certain positions are more comfortable for you or that you need to use a pillow to protect a tender incision or support a part of your body for comfort. Let yourself experiment with ways of pleasuring each other that allow you to feel close without pushing your physical or emotional limits.

For women, the lack of estrogen can make intercourse painful because of the changes in their vaginal lining and lack of natural lubrication. If intercourse causes irritation, use a water-based lubricant or a vaginal suppository. Some women can use an estrogen or testosterone cream to counteract the effects of menopause on their vaginal tissue.

Fertility

Many couples who hope to have children in the future are concerned about how cancer or the cancer-fighting treatments will affect their fertility. This is an important issue to discuss with your doctor. Whether or not it is possible to preserve reproductive functioning depends on a number of things—the kind of cancer you have, your sex and age, as well as the amount, duration, and type of chemotherapy medicines and radiation you receive. In general, every attempt will be made to preserve your fertility without jeopardizing the effectiveness of your treatment. For some people, the effects on fertility will not be known for sure until after all the treatments are over and their body has a chance to return to normal.

Men

The layer of the testes that produces sperm is constantly dividing. Since chemotherapy has the strongest effect on the cells that are frequently dividing, it can have a more detrimental effect on a man's production of sperm than a woman's monthly maturation of a single ovum (egg). When a man receives chemotherapy, his sperm production can decrease or stop altogether. And the sperm that are produced will have less motility, so that they are less able to reach the ovum to fertilize it.

Some chemotherapy medicines are more damaging to fertility than others. If protecting fertility is an important issue, it may be possible to substitute a different drug that will be less damaging to the sperm-producing cells of the testes. As a general rule for chemotherapy, the larger the dose and the longer the period of treatment, the more likely it is that your fertility will be affected.

If it is possible that your treatment may cause infertility, you can consider preserving your sperm in a sperm bank. The sperm is kept frozen for an indefinite period of time. When you want to have a child, the sperm can be thawed and used for artificial insemination of your partner. Preserving your sperm may not be possible if the cancer has caused abnormal sperm or decreased sperm motility. If you are interested in preserving your sperm, ask your doctor or nurse to refer you to a sperm bank in your area where the process is handled in a professional manner, with sensitivity to your feelings and need for privacy.

Women

Even though the ovum-producing layer of the ovary is less damaged by chemotherapy than the testes are, a woman's fertility is still at risk. Chemotherapy often causes menstrual periods to stop during treatment. For women closer to the end of their child-bearing years, their periods may not return even after their treatment is completed, resulting in a premature menopause. As with men, the kind of chemotherapy, dose, and length of treatment are all factors which will influence whether the ovary will continue to produce mature eggs and secrete the hormones necessary for conception.

Women who are facing potential loss of fertility may want to save their eggs or embryos (fertilized eggs) for the future. This process is not as simple as sperm banking. It requires much more time, hormonal stimulation to produce multiple eggs, and more medical intervention. All three of these factors can delay your chemotherapy treatment and recovery. Ask your doctor if you can safely consider this alternative.

Both men and women should continue to use effective birth control during treatment because chemotherapy can damage the ovum, sperm, or the embryo.

Protecting Your Sexuality

If surgery or other cancer treatment will cause changes in your ability to function sexually, even temporarily, you need to know about it ahead of time. Physicians (especially surgeons) recognize their obligation to provide you with enough information so you understand the reason, risks, and alternatives to their recommended treatment. If your regular visits to the oncology office or clinic are too brief to allow you to discuss your concerns, you and your partner can make a "talking appointment" with your physician. Plan a list of questions important to you: How will your ability to enjoy sex be affected? Will it affect your sexual desire? Will your ability to have an erection or orgasm be affected? Does the doctor expect that the problem will be temporary, reversible, or permanent? When will you and your partner be able to resume your normal sexual activities?

If your physician can't answer your questions, he or she may refer you to a specialist for further evaluation. A urologist is a specialist in the urinary tract of both sexes and the genital and reproductive functioning of men. A neurologist is a specialist in diseases involving the nerves and sensations of your body, including the brain and spinal cord. A gynecologist is a specialist in the reproductive function of women. Any of these physician specialists might be helpful in addressing your concerns.

In some cases, short-term sexual counseling with your partner can give both of you the opportunity to explore feelings, fears, and needs around sexuality. A specialist may also be a resource for learning about other positions or means of stimulation that will maximize your enjoyment during this time. Support groups can also be helpful, especially if the group includes others who have had the same kind of cancer or the same kind of cancer-fighting treatment. You may get some ideas about how other couples are dealing with the changes in their sexual lives.

Coping

Your sexuality is not located in any specific organ, nor is it limited to any specific activity. It's much more than that. Your sexuality is a reflection of how you feel about yourself as a man or a woman. It depends in part on your acceptance and appreciation of your body as a source of pleasure to you and your partner. Your sexuality is shaped by your memories and experiences, and it changes all through your life. Because of your illness, you may need to change some of the ways you express your sexuality, but it won't change your need to give and receive some form of loving sexual touch.

Your ability to establish and maintain a sexual connection with someone contributes to the quality of your life. Even though in times of stress or illness having sex may be the last thing on your mind, the need to love and care for another and to be loved and cared for in return is always there. Sexual contact is something that is not only possible during your illness and treatments—it can be a source of comfort, reassurance, passion, and joy.

11

Bone Marrow and Stem-Cell Transplant

You may find the idea of bone marrow and stem-cell transplants a little confusing. When most people think of an organ transplant, they imagine surgery to remove a diseased organ (such as a kidney, liver, or heart), and its replacement with a healthy organ from a donor. You may not consider bone marrow to be an "organ" at all. It's also hard to imagine how someone's diseased bone marrow would be removed, or healthy marrow collected and transplanted to another person. This chapter will give you a general understanding of how bone marrow can be transplanted, and how it can be helpful for some people undergoing cancer-fighting treatments such as chemotherapy and radiation therapy.

What Is Bone Marrow?

Bone marrow is the blood-producing factory of your body. It is tissue within your bones that is capable of producing blood cells (red blood cells, white blood cells, and platelets). As a young child, the marrow in all of your bones was capable of making blood cells. But, as an adult, it is only the marrow of your flat bones like the pelvis, vertebrae, or sternum that is still able to produce these cells. The amount of marrow you have depends on your age and size. The older you are, the less "working" marrow you have.

What Are Stem Cells?

Bone marrow contains a small number of a specialized type of cell called a *stem cell*. The stem cell is capable of dividing and maturing into one of three types of blood cells (red blood cells, white blood cells, or platelets). Under normal conditions, stem cells are continuously dividing and maturing. That is how blood cells are continuously being replaced when they die. When a certain kind of blood cell is needed, the stem cell will start to change into an immature form of that particular cell. When the new blood cell is mature, it is released into the bloodstream.

Stem cells are also sensitive to your body's changing needs in unusual circumstances. For instance, if you have an infection, more of your stem cells will evolve into white blood cells. If you lose a lot of blood because of an accident or surgery, more stem cells will evolve into red blood cells to compensate. Or, if more platelets are needed to form clots, more stem cells will evolve into platelets. Your bone marrow is continuously producing the kinds and amounts of blood cells you need in normal or abnormal conditions.

Not all stem cells are found in the bone marrow. Stem cells also travel in the circulating blood and are called *peripheral* (blood) *stem cells* (PSCs). They are much fewer in number compared to the number of other cells (red blood cells, white blood cells, and platelets) found in circulation. Since chemotherapy and radiation therapy can affect all frequently dividing cells, your bone marrow and the stem cells within it are especially vulnerable to these treatments.

Here are three important facts you should know about bone marrow and peripheral blood stem cells (PSCs):

1. Bone marrow and PSCs can be collected without endangering the donor.

2. Bone marrow and PSCs can be stored for future use.

3. Bone marrow and PSCs can be transplanted to a person whose bone marrow is not functioning. The transplanted marrow or PSCs can eventually grow in the marrow spaces and produce normal blood cells.

Who Might Need a Bone Marrow or Peripheral Stem-Cell (PSC) Transplant?

You may have had chemotherapy in the past and know that the doses and frequencies of the treatment are planned so that normal cells, especially in the bone marrow, can have time to recover. Standard cancer therapy is most often limited by the sensitivity of the bone marrow. The doses and timing of the treatment must allow for the bone marrow to recover, so that normal blood-cell production can continue.

But a bone marrow or a stem-cell transplant makes it possible to get the high-dose therapy without worrying about bone marrow recovery. A patient can get the kind of treatment at the doses necessary to wipe out all cancer cells in the body, even if it means that the blood cell–producing marrow will be destroyed. After the treatment is given, the previously collected PSCs or bone marrow will be transplanted, and the bone marrow will eventually begin to produce normal blood cells again.

A transplant might also be needed if a person has abnormal cells within the bone marrow itself and needs high-dose treatments. In both cases, the high-dose treatments can permanently damage the bone marrow's ability to produce blood cells. After therapy is completed, the damaged bone marrow will need to be replaced by transplanted bone marrow or PSCs so that person can produce blood cells again.

Collecting, Storing, and Transplanting Bone Marrow

Bone marrow looks like blood. It is a dark red liquid that contains stem cells and many red blood cells. Using a needle and syringe, a physician can collect a small amount of bone marrow right in the examination room. The back of the hip bones is the most common area from which to obtain a sample of bone marrow.

This area is fairly close to the body's surface, and it can be numbed with a local anesthetic.

But collecting enough cells for a transplant requires many syringes full of bone marrow. The bone marrow collection (or "harvest") procedure is done in the surgery department where the donor can be given anesthesia. The back and front of the hip bones are good sources for harvesting because these bones usually contain the largest amounts of available bone marrow, and they can be reached without surgery or injury to other organs. The *sternum* (breast bone in the front of the chest where the ribs meet) can also be used to collect bone marrow. No incisions or stitches are needed since only syringes and needles are used by the physician to collect the marrow.

Before the harvest, as in all medical and surgical procedures, the physician and anesthesiologist will review with the donor the possible risks and complications. Usually, once the donor has recovered from the anesthesia, he or she can go home the same day. Because the harvested bone marrow is only a fraction of the donor's total bone marrow, there will still be plenty left to continue making blood cells. The donor's bone marrow will replenish and soon replace the amount that was collected.

The donated marrow contains numerous red blood cells as well as stem cells. Before the collection, donors are usually given medications such as iron or vitamins to increase their red blood cell supply. The donor may also store some of his or her own blood, which can be transfused back afterwards if necessary.

After the harvest, there may be aching and some bruising that will take a few days to go away. The donor should rest and avoid strenuous activity during this period. But since there are no incisions or stitches, the recovery period should be rapid. Most of the time, oral pain medications are enough to relieve the discomfort.

Storing Bone Marrow

The harvested bone marrow is then filtered and processed before being put in IV bags. Since the marrow contains stem cells that must be kept alive, a special preservative is used to prevent stem cell damage. Then the marrow is frozen in liquid nitrogen. The marrow can remain frozen and stored for years until it is used for a transplant.

Transplanting Bone Marrow

After high-dose chemotherapy and/or radiation therapy is completed, the collected bone marrow is given to the patient. If the bone marrow has been frozen and stored, it must be thawed before being given. If the bone marrow is collected from one person and donated immediately to another, it won't be frozen but will be given "fresh" after it is filtered and processed. The marrow, whether thawed or fresh, is given like a blood transfusion into one of the patient's veins (using an IV). Amazingly, the bone marrow cells will migrate from the bloodstream into the patient's bone marrow space where, after a few weeks, it will begin to grow. Then the new marrow can begin to produce blood cells.

Collecting, Storing, and Transplanting Peripheral Stem Cells

Stem cells travel in the circulating blood, but there are far fewer of them compared to the number found in the bone marrow. Even though they are rare, medical science has discovered a way of collecting them from the bloodstream, and using them for a transplant as well. One advantage of collecting stem cells from the circulating blood instead of from the bone marrow is that the donor does not have to undergo a surgical procedure. The collecting is done by a blood-cell separation process called *apheresis* (also known as *pheresis*), which in Greek means "to separate or remove."

When preparing for a PSC collection, the donor will be given a medication to send more stem cells from the marrow out into the blood circulation. The more stem cells circulating in the blood, the faster they can be collected by pheresis.

The pheresis machine looks similar to the kind used for kidney dialysis. An IV is inserted in the donor's arm, and his or her blood flows through IV tubing into the machine. The blood circulates through the machine, which spins the blood to separate out the stem cells. Then the blood is returned to the donor through another IV tube that has been inserted in the donor's other arm. Blood continues to circulate from the donor, through the pheresis machine, and back to the donor in a continuous loop. Approximately one cup of blood is circulating through the machine at any time. Since there are so few stem cells in circulation, the collection process may take three to six hours a day for several days to collect enough stem cells for a transplant.

If the veins in the donor's arms are not large enough to be used for the pheresis collection, the physician may insert an IV catheter in one of the larger veins of the upper chest or groin. The catheter has two IV tubes fused together, so one tube can be used for blood flowing out from the donor into the pheresis machine, and the other can be used for blood flowing back to the donor. This catheter is taken out as soon as enough stem cells have been collected and the pheresis procedure is finished. The collected stem cells, like bone marrow, can be preserved and frozen. They are either stored for future use or transplanted shortly after collection.

Following high-dose chemotherapy and/or radiation therapy, the collected PSCs are given to the recipient intravenously, like a blood transfusion. And just like transplanted bone marrow, the stem cells will migrate to the bone marrow spaces. Once the stem cells start to grow in the marrow spaces, they can begin producing normal blood cells.

Two Kinds of Transplants

There are two types of bone marrow and peripheral stem-cell transplants. They are distinguished by whether you are donating to yourself, or receiving marrow or peripheral stem cells from a donor.

Autologous Transplant

When bone marrow or peripheral stem cells taken from a patient are given back to that same patient following high-dose therapy, this is called an *autologous transplant*. "Auto" comes from the Greek word meaning "self," and an autologous transplant is, in effect, a transplant to yourself.

Many patients who receive an autologous transplant may have perfectly normal bone marrow. But because standard anticancer treatments may not be adequate to eliminate all the cancer, high-dose chemotherapy and/or radiation therapy may be considered. These high-dose treatments, while killing the cancer, can also destroy the blood-producing capacity of the bone marrow. Therefore, bone marrow or peripheral stem cells are collected and stored before high-dose therapy begins so that it can be given back to that same person after the treatments are completed.

Other patients who receive an autologous transplant may not have normal bone marrow. For example, diseases such as acute leukemia or some kinds of lymphoma affect the marrow's ability to produce healthy blood cells. Chemotherapy can wipe out the abnormal cells, at least temporarily. During the time that the marrow is free of detectable disease, the bone marrow or peripheral stem cells can be collected and stored. Then treatment can continue using high-dose therapy, followed by an autologous transplant. Or, after the marrow or PSCs are stored, the person has the option of waiting. If the disease returns, the person can have high-dose therapy to treat the disease, followed by an autologous transplant.

Allogeneic Transplant

When the transplanted bone marrow or peripheral stem cells come from another person, it is called an *allogeneic transplant.* The word "allo" comes from the Greek word meaning "other."

A person may have diseased marrow that cannot be cleared, even temporarily, of abnormal cells by conventional chemotherapy or radiation therapy. That person will depend on a donor to provide him or her with new bone marrow or PSCs in order to reestablish blood-cell production. After high-dose therapy clears the marrow spaces, the donated marrow cells or PSCs are given by IV to the recipient. The donated cells then migrate from the bloodstream to the bone marrow space, where they grow and produce healthy blood cells.

The Importance of a Close Match

The donor (the person giving the marrow or PSCs) must have marrow that is a very close match to the recipient's. If it is not a close match, the donated marrow may not grow in the marrow spaces—it will be rejected.

The bone marrow is part of the immune system. It is supposed to help fight against anything that does not belong in the body (like bacteria or viruses). With an allogeneic transplant, the marrow did not come from the recipient, but from another person. If the new marrow is not a very close match to the recipient's, it may identify the recipient's cells as being foreign. It may produce immune cells that attack the recipient's cells and organs. This creates a condition known as *graft vs. host disease* or GVHD. The "graft" is the donated marrow; the "host" is the person receiving the donated marrow. There is more information about how to prevent and treat GVHD later in this chapter.

How a Donor Is Chosen

The perfect donor for an allogeneic bone marrow transplant would be an identical twin, since both twins come from the same genetic material. For most people, that is not an option. You may, however, find a close match in your immediate family such as a sibling, parent, or a more distant relative. Less frequently, a match may be found with an unrelated donor. Potential donors have their blood tested, and if the first tests show a possible match, more blood tests are done to assure compatibility. Potential donors do not need to have their bone marrow tested.

From a blood sample, the recipient's genetic material (DNA and chromosomes) is compared to the potential donor's to see how closely they are matched. The lab may even mix the recipient's lymphocytes (an important part of the immune system) with those of the potential donor's to see if they will attack each other. Careful testing of potential donors reduces the chances of the recipient developing GVHD or rejecting the new marrow. Potential donors are also tested for diseases such as hepatitis or AIDS which might be passed on to the recipient along with the new marrow cells or PSCs during the transplant.

Deciding on a Treatment Plan

Your doctor will recommend a treatment plan after considering many factors—the kind of cancer you have, the types of cancer-fighting treatments you have had in the past, and your response to those treatments. He or she will also consider your age, physical condition, the availability of donors, and so on. Transplant centers throughout the world share information, so your physician will know what treatments have been successful for similar patients. However, there may be more than one way to treat your type of disease, and having a transplant is just one option. Your doctor will discuss the recommended treatment plan with you.

The Pretransplant Phase

In addition to your transplant doctor, you and your family will meet with a number of people in the "transplant team." Besides the oncologist and nurses, the team may include a nurse coordinator, nutritionist, social worker, pharmacist, physical therapist, and others who will be involved in your care. The team will also work with your insurance company to get authorization for the transplant. This may require special documentation, additional tests, second opinions, or other appeals to show that bone marrow or PSC transplant is an appropriate and effective treatment for your disease.

This is the time for you to ask questions, to get an understanding of the risks and benefits of the treatment, the different phases of the transplant procedure, and about how long each phase can be expected to last. You may have the chance to talk to someone who has gone through a similar procedure and who can share his or her experience with you.

During the pretransplant phase, your doctor will reevaluate your physical condition, rechecking your heart, lungs, liver, and kidneys. You will also be tested for previous exposure to diseases such as hepatitis, herpes, and other viruses, because some viral diseases could become reactivated once treatment begins and your immune system is not functioning.

Insertion of a Central Venous Catheter

During the transplant period, you will need IV medications, chemotherapy, fluids, nutrition, blood products, antibiotics, and many blood tests. A central catheter is an IV catheter similar to the ones that are used in your arms, but it is inserted into a large vein in your upper chest or neck. It provides the doctors and nurses immediate and continuous access to your blood system without having to use the narrower veins of your hands or arms. All medications, fluids, chemotherapy, and blood products can be give through this catheter, swept along in the rapid blood flow near the heart. Blood for most lab tests can also be taken painlessly from the central catheter.

The central catheter used during a transplant is made so that two or more catheters are actually fused together into one tube. Once in place, it looks like a single catheter as it comes through the skin, but the end of the catheter splits off into two or more "tails." These tails can be attached to separate IV infusions. This enables the nurses to give you different medications at the same time and draw blood for lab tests as well. See Chapter 4 ("The IV Experience") for more descriptions and illustrations of central catheters.

Standard Chemotherapy Prior to High-Dose Therapy

Your doctor may recommend one or more treatments of standard-dose chemotherapy to treat your disease before collecting bone marrow or peripheral stem cells. There are a number of reasons for this. First, your doctor wants to see if the chemotherapy is effective in killing the cancer cells. Second, your doctor may want to eliminate as much of the cancer as possible before the transplant. Third, the chemotherapy will eventually produce an increase in the number of stem cells both in the bone marrow and in the blood circulation. (After chemotherapy, there is a temporary slow-down in blood cell production. But when the bone marrow recovers it produces a surge in the number of stem cells.) These circulating PSCs are then collected by pheresis for the transplant.

High-Dose Therapy—Conditioning

The *conditioning regimen* is the combination of high-dose treatments you will receive in an attempt to wipe out all the cancer cells in the body. This high-dose treatment may contain chemotherapy drugs, or it may combine chemotherapy and radiation therapy. The conditioning regimen is similar to a "recipe" for treatment.

Nausea is an immediate side effect of the high-dose therapy, so you will be given anti-nausea medications to prevent this problem. Other side effects of the treatment, such as clearing the bone marrow, hair loss, changes in mucous membranes of your mouth and digestive system, diarrhea, and skin changes, will become evident over the next few weeks.

Total Body Irradiation (TBI)

Standard radiation treatments usually direct the radiation to a limited area. Organs and tissues surrounding the tumor are shielded to minimize radiation exposure outside the treatment field. With TBI, your whole body will be exposed to a level of radiation that will help eradicate all cancer cells while not causing permanent damage to normal cells.

One purpose of TBI is to destroy all cancer cells even if they have spread to distant areas and even if they are not detectable on scans or other tests. For those patients receiving bone marrow or stem cells from a donor (allogeneic transplant), TBI helps to clear out the old marrow space so the new marrow can move in more easily and start producing blood cells.

Not all transplant patients will receive high-dose radiation as part of their treatment plan. It will depend on a number of factors including the kind of cancer you have, whether or not the cancer is sensitive to radiation, whether or not you have had radiation treatments in the past, and so on. If your doctor recommends TBI as part of your conditioning regimen, you will go for treatments once or twice a day for a few days, in conjunction with the high-dose chemotherapy.

The exact radiation dose will be calculated carefully by a radiation oncologist to ensure that the dose of radiation you receive is the same throughout your body. Sometimes only the lymph tissue (lymph nodes and spleen) is irradiated and the rest of the body is shielded. This is called *total lymphoid irradiation* (TLI). If radiation therapy is part of your treatment plan, the radiation oncologist will explain more about it to you, as well as the risks, benefits, and side effects you might experience.

As with chemotherapy, an immediate side effect of TBI is often nausea. You will be given antinausea medication to prevent this problem. A nurse will be with you when you go for the treatment in the radiation oncology department to make sure you are comfortable and the antinausea medications are working. Although you will be alone in the room during the several minutes of treatment, you will be watched via a monitor. When the treatment is over, you can return to your room.

The Transplant—"Day 0"

The day you receive the marrow or peripheral stem cells is called "Day 0." Every day after the transplant is then numbered to keep track of when certain medicines are given and how long it takes until blood cells are produced by the new marrow. If you received TBI first, followed by high-dose chemotherapy, you will have a few days of rest while the last traces of these medications are cleared from your body. If your chemotherapy was followed by TBI, you may receive the transplant as soon as the radiation treatments are completed.

On the day of the transplant, the bone marrow or peripheral stem cells are brought to your room in small IV bags. First, you will be given medications to prevent an allergic reaction to the cells or the preservative in which the cells are stored. Your nurse will stay with you and monitor you continuously (watching your temperature, blood pressure, and so on). He or she will help you to stay warm, relaxed, and comfortable. If the marrow or PSCs are to be given on the same day as they were collected, they will be infused just like a blood transfusion over a few hours.

If the marrow or PSCs have been frozen, the nurse or technician will thaw each bag, one at a time, in a warm-water bath. After each bag is thawed, it will be given through the IV very quickly. If there are many bags of frozen PSCs to be infused, you may not get them all at once. To prevent you from getting overloaded with too much fluid or preservative, you may get the transplant in two or more sessions.

Once infused, the marrow or PSCs will migrate to the bone marrow spaces where they will grow and eventually begin to produce blood cells.

The Recovery Period

The transplanted marrow or stem cells will begin to produce blood cells in about one to four weeks, although it will take longer for your immune system to recover completely. The high-dose cancer-fighting treatments you received have hopefully destroyed cancer cells all through your body. Your normal cells, especially those cells that divide frequently, will need time to recover. The rapidly dividing cells of your digestive system, mucous membranes, and hair follicles are especially affected.

Until your marrow starts to produce blood cells, you will need intensive monitoring and expert medical and nursing care. This may include the following:

- Multiple transfusions to replace red blood cells and platelets when needed

- Antibiotics and other medications to fight infections

- IV pain medication if you have discomfort from mouth sores or abdominal cramping

- Medications to prevent and relieve nausea, vomiting, and diarrhea

- IV fluids and IV nutrition if you are unable to eat or drink adequately

- A meticulous mouth care program to keep the mucous membranes of your mouth clean and disinfected in order to prevent infection and promote healing

- Frequent skin care to keep all your skin clean and lubricated in order to prevent infections or discomfort.

You will also need support from all the members of the transplant team—your physicians and nurses, the nutritionist, physical therapist, respiratory therapist, and social worker, among others. The support of your family and close friends is also very important. They provide things that no one else can—a familiar face, a comforting presence, distraction, humor, and a connection to home.

Replacing Red Blood Cells and Platelets

The day you receive your bone marrow or PSC transplant (Day 0), you will, of course, still have blood cells circulating in your bloodstream. The mature blood cells already in circulation do not divide, so they are relatively unaffected by the high-dose chemotherapy and radiation treatments. But blood cells do not live forever—they need to be replaced continuously. For a time, your marrow will be unable to produce new cells as it normally does.

Your daily blood test will show your blood counts dropping as the cells in circulation die off. Until your new bone marrow begins to function, you may need transfusions to provide you with red blood cells (the cells that carry oxygen from your lungs to every part of your body) and platelets (the cells that help stop bleeding by forming clots). Since platelets live only eight to ten days, you will need platelet transfusions most frequently—sometimes more than once a day. Red blood cells live longer (about 120 days), but you will probably need transfusions of those cells as well.

While you are waiting for the new bone marrow to begin functioning, you may also be given daily injections of a hormone that will stimulate the stem cells in the bone marrow to begin to divide and grow into white cells as soon as possible. You would get either G-CSF (Granulocyte Colony Stimulating Factor) or GM-CSF (Granulocyte-Macrophage Colony Stimulating Factor). By encouraging the early return of these white blood cells, the injections shorten the period of time when you are most susceptible to infection.

Many people have concerns about blood transfusions because they worry about the risk of contracting the AIDS virus (HIV) or hepatitis from contaminated blood. Years ago, when there were no effective tests to identify contaminated blood, it certainly was a serious risk. But now all blood is screened to greatly reduce the risk of transmitting these diseases to the people receiving blood transfusions.

You do have the option of asking family members and friends with compatible blood to donate for you. But during the immediate recovery period you may need so many transfusions, it can be difficult lining up enough designated donors that qualify to donate blood. Many potential blood donors may be disqualified because of their age, weight, general health, history of previous infections, or if they take certain medications. Your transplant coordinator will give you more information about this if you are interested in having designated donors provide red blood cells and platelets during this time.

Preventing Infections

While your immune system is recovering, prevention and treatment of infections is most important. Infections can be caused by organisms in your outer environment as well as organisms that live on or in your body (i.e., skin or digestive tract). Everything possible will be done to prevent exposure to any source of infection. And if you show any sign of infection (fever, diarrhea, pain, redness, and so on), it will be treated with appropriate medications to fight it.

Depending on your transplant center, you may be in the hospital for your entire transplant period from the first high-dose treatments to recovery. Some transplant centers provide certain patients the option of having the transplant as an outpatient. If you were to get treatment as an outpatient, you would most likely come to the clinic every day for treatment and testing and then go home at night. The decision about outpatient treatment will depend on your transplant center, the availability of someone to help you at home, the recommendation of your physician, and the transplant team.

There is some variation in how strictly isolated you will be during the time you are waiting for your immune system to recover. Some centers have special isolation rooms for transplant patients, with an air filtration system to filter out some of the organisms that can cause infections. Other transplant centers have rooms that attempt to provide a totally sterile environment, with filtered air, masks, and sterile clothing for anyone entering the room.

No matter what your environment (at home or in the hospital), certain precautions are always taken to protect you from infections. Everyone who comes to see you—doctors, nurses, housekeepers, visitors, and so on—should wash their hands with an antibacterial soap before entering your room or touching you. In the hospital, no plants or fresh flowers are allowed in the room since they can harbor bacteria. You will be on a low-bacteria diet. Some transplant centers will only allow you to eat well cooked foods and drink sterile water. Other centers allow you to eat some fresh fruits and vegetables and drink the tap water. Your transplant team will let you know what restrictions are recommended in the hospital or at home.

Controlling outside sources of infection is half the battle. Your body surfaces also carry many organisms that can cause infections when your immunity is temporarily impaired. During this time, you will need to shower daily with an antibacterial soap and wash carefully after each time you use the toilet. You will be cleansing your mouth several times a day and rinsing with an antibacterial mouthwash. The place where your central catheter comes out of your skin (or any open area on your skin) will be carefully observed to check for any signs of infection, and the area will be disinfected and covered with a sterile dressing.

Medications are an essential weapon in fighting infections. Until your bone marrow begins to produce white blood cells again, infections can be deadly. You may be started on antibiotics before your white blood cell count drops. With any sign of an infection, your nurse will get a sample of your blood or other secretions (urine, stool, sputum, etc.) so the lab can identify the exact organism causing the infection and determine an effective medication to eliminate it. Even before the organism is identified you will probably be given antibiotics that can kill a broad range of bacteria. If you have had herpes or chicken pox in the past, right from the start you may also be given an anti-viral medication (like acyclovir) to prevent reactivation of those diseases.

Preventing Nausea and Vomiting

During the days when you were getting the high-dose cancer-fighting therapy, you received medicine to prevent nausea and vomiting. For some patients, nausea can continue to be a problem even after the high-dose therapy is completed. They may feel nauseated even if they are not eating anything. If this occurs, they will continue to take antinausea medicines for as long as they are needed. There are many different kinds of medications available that work in different ways to relieve nausea. Chapter 5 ("Coping with Nausea") has more information about the medications used to prevent and relieve nausea.

Mouth and Throat Pain

We tend to think of the digestive system as a series of organs— Mouth, esophagus, stomach, intestines, and so on. But, in reality, your digestive system is one long tube. Digestion starts in your mouth when you chew your food and mix it with saliva. Food goes down your esophagus to the stomach and then to the small intestine, where digestion continues and nutrients are absorbed. The large intestine is the place where fluid is absorbed back into circulation.

The entire digestive tube is lined with cells which are frequently dividing. These cells wear out and are constantly replaced by new cells. Since chemotherapy and radiation therapy causes a delay in the production of new cells, the entire digestive system from beginning to end is affected.

About a week after your high-dose therapy, the loss of the cells lining your mouth may cause the mucous membranes of your mouth—gums, inner cheeks, pallet, lips, and throat—to become raw and painful. Even if you have done the most careful mouth care, you can still develop mouth sores. These sores may be so painful that you need IV pain medication to relieve the pain, and IV fluids and nutrition until you can eat normally again.

The temporary loss of cells lining your mouth leaves you susceptible to infection. You need to clean and disinfect your mouth every few hours to prevent infection and promote healing. Mucous membranes that are clean and moist heal faster. The new lining of mucous membranes will return in a few weeks, about the time your bone marrow begins to produce blood cells again.

Diarrhea

After the high-dose therapy and transplant, you may experience diarrhea or frequent, loose stools. Just as in your mouth or throat, the lining of the rest of the digestive system will also be lost. This may cause temporary sores and oozing of blood in your intestines, which can be very irritating to your bowels. You may experience diarrhea and cramping pain as your digestive tract speeds up in an attempt to get rid of the irritation. Diarrhea can cause severe loss of essential fluids and chemicals (electrolytes) if it is not controlled. Daily blood tests help your doctor monitor and replace fluids and electrolytes (like potassium or sodium) that you need while you are having diarrhea.

Infection in the intestines can also cause diarrhea and cramping. To check if you have an infection, a sample of your stool will be sent to the lab for testing. There are a number of organisms that can infect the bowel. One of them, *clostridia difficile*, produces a toxin. Diarrhea can be caused by the body's attempt to get rid of this toxin. If you have "C-Diff" toxin in your stool, you will first be given medicine to eradicate the infection that is producing the toxin, and then medicine to stop the diarrhea.

Engraftment

Engraftment is the term used to describe the point in time, after the transplant, when the new bone marrow begins to produce blood cells. Because you have been getting transfusions of red blood cells and platelets after the transplant, it's hard to tell when the bone marrow starts producing these cells. The first sign that blood-cell production has resumed is that your daily blood test will show the presence of white blood cells. This means engraftment has occurred.

Once your bone marrow begins to function, you will start to feel better. Mouth sores and sores in the digestive tract will begin to heal, and mouth pain, nausea, and diarrhea will abate. As your immune system kicks in, you will have fewer fevers and begin to feel more energy. Once the mouth sores are healed and you are feeling less nausea, you will begin to eat and drink again and need less IV fluid and nutritional support. When your bone marrow has adequate numbers of red blood cells and platelets, you will no longer need transfusions. Eventually you'll no longer need IV antibiotics as your immune system returns to normal. If you have been in the hospital for the transplant period, you will be discharged home.

Graft-Versus-Host Disease (GVHD)

GVHD is a complication that can develop after an allogeneic transplant (the transplanted bone marrow or stem cells came from another person). It rarely develops after an autologous transplant since the recipient receives his own bone marrow or stem cells. It occurs when the transplanted marrow from the donor (the graft) starts to function as part of the immune system. When the immune system tries to fight off foreign invaders, the transplanted cells attack the host's cells, reading them as foreign.

GVHD can affect any part of the body, and varies from mild to severe. It most commonly affects the skin, liver, or digestive system. Skin GVHD appears initially as a fine red rash that is usually seen on the torso, hands, and feet. Later, the skin GVHD can appear as a dark thickening of the skin. GVHD of the digestive tract will cause large amounts of diarrhea. Blood tests can indicate early signs of liver damage due to GVHD. Since there are many other things that can cause rashes, diarrhea, or changes in liver function, these symptoms do not necessarily indicate the disease.

In many cases, GVHD can be prevented. Selection of a compatible donor is the first step. The closer the match, the less likely GVHD will develop. Sometimes the collected bone marrow or PSCs are treated before they are transplanted so that the new immune system is less likely to cause GVHD.

Prevention and Treatment of GVHD. Even before the transplant, the recipient of an allogeneic transplant will begin to take an immuno-suppressive medicine to prevent GVHD. A drug commonly prescribed is cyclosporine A. This is usually given once or twice a day, and you will continue to take it for many months after the transplant.

Side effects of cyclosporin A include high blood pressure, increased hair growth, and kidney problems. People who take this medication may notice an increase in hair growth, on the head as well as on the face. They may also need to take medication to lower their blood pressure while taking cyclosporine A. Since this drug can cause kidney damage, it is especially important to drink a lot of fluids. That will prevent dehydration, keep a good blood flow to your kidneys, and help protect them from the potentially damaging effects of cyclosporine A. The dose of this drug may change depending on your symptoms. The doctor will be testing your blood frequently and adjusting the dose so it is most effective to prevent the disease, without causing serious side effects.

Another medication used to prevent GVHD is the steroid prednisone. Prednisone is usually started a few weeks after the transplant and may be continued for several months. Side effects of prednisone can include weight gain, mood shifts, feeling very "wired," insomnia, and upset stomach. Steroids such as prednisone can also cause an elevation in the blood sugar. If you are diabetic, this may mean that you will have to adjust your blood sugar medications while taking prednisone.

Since prednisone can cause problems sleeping, it is recommended that you take it early in the day rather than at bed time. Prednisone may also irritate your stomach or cause ulcers. Always take prednisone along with food. Medications that decrease stomach acid production such as Prilosec, Zantac, or Pepcid can also be helpful.

Another drug often given to prevent GVHD is methotrexate. Larger doses of methotrexate are used with other chemotherapy drugs to kill cancer cells. When given in several small doses in the immediate posttransplant phase, methotrexate suppresses the immune system and prevents GVHD. Side effects may include nausea, mouth sores, and slightly delayed engraftment.

If you had an allogeneic transplant, you will continue taking GVHD medications for many months. Sometimes, even if you have been taking the medication faithfully, you may still develop GVHD. If this happens, your doctor may change the medication or the dose to control the problem. After your allogeneic transplant, your physician and nurses will be following you very carefully, checking your blood tests and monitoring your symptoms to identify and treat GVHD at an early stage if it develops.

Back to Normal

Full recovery after a transplant is a gradual process. At first you may continue to have some nausea and diarrhea, and your appetite may be slow to return. You may still have intermittent fevers, or you may need to continue getting fluids, antibiotics, and blood transfusions for several weeks. You may still feel fragile and fatigued. During this time you will be closely monitored by your physician and nurses in the clinic and in your home. You'll be given instructions about your diet, medications, and mouth and skin care. But each week will bring you closer to feeling like your normal self. Soon your appetite and energy (and hair) will return. You'll spend less time at the clinic and more time doing the activities of your normal life.

Emotional recovery is also a gradual process. While people are going through the transplant and early recovery period, their focus is necessarily on the immediate physical challenges of managing symptoms, watching blood counts, taking medications—survival. Their attention has been on getting through each day, sometimes each hour. While they are undergoing treatment, they can feel totally removed from their regular world of job, family, and social activities. With recovery, there is a gradual change in focus. If you were in the hospital for the transplant, you may feel anxiety about going home where you will not have medical help and nursing support twenty-four hours a day.

It may take a while to "digest" all that you've experienced. Your family, friends, and medical team may have been with you during the transplant, but they have not been through it. If your hospital or clinic sponsors a support group for posttransplant patients, you might find it helpful to attend. You might also find it helpful to talk to another "graduate" who has been through it. Or you may find it helpful to meet with a counselor who is familiar with the emotional issues that come up during this time. Over the weeks, your strength and stamina will return, and you'll feel less fragile in the "real world" both physically and emotionally.

In Summary

Your transplant center may do some things differently than what is described in this chapter. That's inevitable, because this procedure is constantly evolving. Medications and techniques are changing quickly. Hopefully, new medications and techniques will continue to improve this treatment by shortening the period of time it takes for the bone marrow to begin to produce blood cells, and by preventing the serious side effects. What's important to remember is that bone marrow and peripheral stem cell transplants offer many people a chance of cure when standard therapies would not have been as effective.

12

Mind and Body
by Burton A. Presberg, M.D.

I listen to people tell stories about their lives and cancer. They talk about their families, jobs, and living situations. They tell how cancer has profoundly changed their lives. Cancer affects much more than bodies. Life itself is suddenly different in almost every way. Previous chapters have detailed many of the physical aspects of cancer and its treatment; this chapter focuses on the mental and emotional. This chapter is about you, the human being who happens to have gotten this disease.

The chapter is divided into four sections. The first is about emotions. You may be experiencing a whole range of feelings; this first section is about understanding and accepting them. The next section addresses the connection between mind and body—what we know and don't know in this controversial area. The third section focuses on methods to help you cope, live, and feel better. These include counseling, support groups, religion and spirituality, and other complementary therapies. The final section provides some hints in finding the path that is right for you.

Dealing with cancer is difficult and challenging. It can feel awful and unfair. Nevertheless, you can use your strengths and the support of others to cope to the best of your ability. The obstacles on the journey are many—hopefully this chapter will provide you with some strategies to maneuver through them.

Living with Cancer

The Trauma of Diagnosis

Receiving a cancer diagnosis is extremely traumatic. This is true regardless of the type of cancer, its stage, or whether the diagnosis was expected or unexpected. A variety of emotions may emerge, and these feelings may stay constant or change repeatedly. You may feel like screaming or crying, or you may feel engulfed in a fog. The shock may alternate with numbness, in which you may feel nothing or even "forget" you have cancer. Then cancer suddenly jumps back into your awareness and you feel scared, angry, and overwhelmed. You may recognize your emotions as being similar to an experience of losing a loved one or receiving other devastating news. This back-and-forth shows the struggle your mind is having with accepting unwanted news. Minds work this way. You are not going crazy, even though it may feel like it at times.

Initial shock is often followed by a period of activity. This is the time to learn more about the illness and treatment options. You gather your strength, identify your supports, and make necessary work and home arrangements. This is a period of rearranging priorities, determining what is really important to you, and perhaps learning to appreciate little things more. This may well be the period that you are in now, as you read this book.

Your Emotions

Fear, anger, and sadness are some of the many emotions you may be feeling. These responses may be very difficult to accept, particularly if you are used to feeling in control. In addition to your body not acting as you would like, your emotions are running out of control. Treatment and its side effects, particularly fatigue, sleeplessness, and nausea, add to these mood swings.

It is very important to understand that all of this is *normal*. Simply allowing yourself to have all of these feelings is a crucial step. Of course, everyone differs in their degree of comfort in expressing emotions, but, as much as possible, let it out. You may wish to do it by yourself, with friends and loved ones, or with a therapist or support group.

The necessity of thinking positively is a myth. The whole spectrum of emotions, from negative to positive, is unavoidable and necessary. Not letting yourself feel how you feel, or getting upset at yourself for being angry or sad, can backfire and cause you to feel even worse that you did before. On the other hand, a good cry or yell often is relieving and healing. Feelings provide us with vital information. Denying them or keeping them inside may in fact be the unhealthy choice.

Your mind may continue to fight the truth at times, but eventually reality sets in. The cancer exists and however much you dream and wish for its sudden disappearance, the struggle continues, at least for now. Accepting reality does not mean being passive. Instead it means doing everything you can do to help yourself, while at the same time learning to live with what cannot be changed. You will learn to live your life with cancer, perhaps in better ways than you ever expected. A shift often takes place, a shift from feeling like a victim, from feeling "why me," to feeling that living the best you can with your illness is a challenge and a motivation.

Sadness Is Okay—Depression Is Not

Having cancer is undeniably difficult, physically and emotionally. Sadness is expected; it is normal and inevitable. The feeling of sadness is often called depression, but clinical depression (also called major depression) is entirely different. Clinical depression is a reversible illness. It extends beyond normal sadness to cloud every aspect of the sufferer's existence. In a physically healthy person, problems with sleeping, eating, and maintaining energy will point toward a diagnosis of clinical depression. In a person with cancer, difficulties in these areas are almost universal; therefore they cannot be used to determine whether a person has depression.

Distinguishing normal sadness from clinical depression in a person who has cancer depends on psychological symptoms. A person with cancer feels sad, but still feels that he or she is a good person. A person with clinical depression has a poor self-image. A sad person can still enjoy activities and relationships;

someone with depression loses the ability to feel pleasure and often withdraws from family and friends. A sad person maintains a balanced view of the world and feels capable of doing things to help himself. A person with clinical depression often feels the entire world is hopeless and that he or she is entirely helpless and unable to change any aspect of the situation. While a sad person may think about death, a person with depression dwells on death and often has suicidal thoughts.

Identifying clinical depression is important because it is treatable. Treatment includes counseling and often an antidepressant medication such as Prozac, Paxil, Zoloft, Desyrel, or Wellbutrin. Medications often take a number of weeks to work, but over time, mood and outlook usually improve significantly. Side effects, particularly with the newer antidepressants, are generally minimal. Antidepressants work by raising the level of certain chemicals in the brain. These chemicals (called *neurotransmitters*) stabilize mood and control anxiety. The goal is to help you feel like yourself, undoubtedly dealing with a difficult situation, but still the same person underneath. Antidepressants do not block feelings of sadness or take away your feelings, nor do they cause dependence.

If you feel you may be suffering from depression, please speak with your doctor. You or you doctor may wish to consult with a mental health professional about counseling. Consultation with a psychiatrist about medication is also a possibility, though any physician can prescribe antidepressants.

Family and Friends

This is a time in your life when, more than ever, you need the support of family and friends. You need concrete physical support, such as help with medical paperwork, transportation, and housework. You also need emotional support: someone to listen and provide a shoulder to cry on.

Asking for support is not always easy. You may not want to bother anyone, or you may worry about having your privacy invaded by an army of helpers. It is particularly hard for those of us who are used to giving aid, rather than being aided. It is a slow, step-by-step process to get comfortable asking for help. A useful way to look at this is that, in most cases, others *want* to be there for you. This allows them to feel useful and needed during a difficult time for everyone. Allowing others to be supportive can really be your way of helping them—allowing them in rather that shutting them out.

Be patient with yourself and those around you. Be clear with others about what you need and don't need. Don't expect others to be able to read your mind. Having cancer can significantly change relationships, roles, and responsibilities. During treatment you may not be able to pull your own weight at home or at work, and it is going to take time and effort to reassign responsibilities. Resentments may come up, as well as old fights you thought were long behind you. Open discussion and communication have never been more important.

Mind and Body: What's the Connection?

The relationship between the mind and the body has been debated throughout human history. Our ancestors had no doubt of the connection, and ancient rituals were designed to heal mind and body together. The rise of medical science in this century led to the opposite viewpoint, the view that mind and body are split and unrelated. Medical science has focused on cells, chemicals, CAT scans and other measurable physical realities. Recently the pendulum has begun to swing back, and many are preaching the unity of mind and body. Whom should you believe?

The Appeal and Limitations of Mind/Body Unity

At the basic level there is no doubt that mind and body are inextricably connected. Blushing from embarrassment or nervous butterflies in the stomach remind you of this reality. Fear causes goosebumps. Research has clearly demonstrated the connection between a Type A personality and heart disease. But what does this mean for the person with cancer? The truth is somewhere in the middle. Mind and body undoubtedly interact and work together. But the details of the connection are not clear and are often overstated. This in itself can be dangerous, leading to guilt over having "caused" your illness and feeling extraordinary pressure to heal yourself.

Certainly living a happy, stress-free life while keeping a positive attitude is admirable, but, for most of us, it's much more easily said than done. The problem is that you may feel pressured to make changes in your life that are unrealistic and unattainable. The mind may account for *some* changes in the body, but you certainly cannot be expected to heal your cancer simply by thinking it away. The mind controls the body to some extent, but certainly not completely.

Unfortunately, cancer is a powerful biological illness. The mind/body advocates are tapping into a universal human wish—the desire to have control of one's own life and destiny. It's no wonder that people flock to any approach that promises a cure. The downside comes when the mind/body approaches do not succeed in curing.

Dangers: Guilt, Responsibility, and Quackery

The mind/body approaches may lead to feelings of guilt or responsibility. Guilt may arise if you are unable to will away your cancer. Oversubscribing to mind/body views can put too much responsibility on your already burdened shoulders, weight you may not be willing to bear. It is one thing to work together with your doctor to do what can be done; it is another to feel that all of a sudden you have to change everything about the way you think, feel, and relate to the world.

Quackery is a significant danger. Unfortunately, many prey on those who are willing to consider anything that can provide a sense of hope and control. Investigate alternative methods carefully and run, don't walk, away from anyone who promises a cure. The risk is losing a lot of money, or worse, physical endangerment from untested methodologies that conflict with or interact adversely with other medical care. While physicians vary in their views of these alternative therapies, it is crucial to talk with yours to find out if there are specific risks to your health.

You Did Not Ask for Cancer

This is a crucial point. Even if you have lung cancer clearly related to smoking, you did not intend to get the disease. It is also crucial to understand that despite suggestions that depression, anxiety, stress, or personality can cause cancer, there is no good scientific evidence to prove this. Everyone has anxiety and stress in their lives, so it is easy for someone who gets cancer to imagine that it was caused by these things. Some of the calmest, happiest people get cancer, and some of the most depressed, stressed-out people never get cancer. Blaming yourself for your illness is unnecessary, unproductive, and most importantly, untrue.

It is understandable that you would try to find a reason for your cancer. People want things to make sense. We want there to be an explanation for why things happen. Unfortunately, with cancer there often is no satisfactory explanation. Sometimes things just happen, with no rhyme or reason. Justice and fairness do not always prevail.

Where All This Leaves You

The bottom line is this: mind and body work both together and separately. The connection is real, but not absolute. Addressing where your mind, thoughts, and emotions are during this experience is important for its own sake. Your mind creates your perception of reality and your experience of your life. Respect the profound importance of this, but do not take it too far.

Practically speaking, this means doing what feels right to you. It means accepting the unknown and realizing there are no guarantees. Take care of both your mind and your body as best as you can. If visualizing white blood cells fighting cancer feels right to you, do it. If it doesn't, spend your time in other ways.

The challenge is being at the same time open-minded to new ideas and approaches, yet skeptical. The key is clarity of purpose. If used to improve well-being and quality of life, a number of mind/body approaches can be very useful. If, on the other hand, the goal is to cure cancer, trouble may arise.

Help Along the Way

There is plenty of help available. Struggling with cancer, its treatment, and your own feelings is not something you have to do alone. The approaches are numerous and varied. This section introduces some of the possible avenues you may wish to pursue to help you cope and live your life with cancer.

Individual Counseling

Talking to a therapist is an option to consider. You are going through a lot right now, both physically and emotionally. Talking with family and friends can be very helpful. Still, it is very different to talk to an objective outsider. A therapist or counselor does not have personal ties to you, so the relationship exists entirely for you. You may feel the need to comfort and soothe your loved ones and may not wish to subject them to all of your sad, angry, or other difficult feelings. With a therapist, you can let it all hang out. Simply verbalizing feelings out loud to another person can be comforting and freeing.

It is important to find a therapist who has experience in working with people with cancer. Your medical system may have designated support people, or your doctors or nurses may have practitioners they have referred to before. The type of therapist is not as important as finding someone you feel comfortable talking to. You will want to seek out an M.D. (psychiatrist) if medication issues are likely to be involved, but otherwise, a Ph.D. psychologist, a masters-level counselor, or a social worker are all possibilities.

Make sure you and your therapist are clear on the goals and process of therapy. Sessions may be scheduled on an as-needed basis or scheduled more regularly, such as once a week or once every two weeks. Clarify the type of therapy you want and need. Therapy can focus on bolstering your existing coping mechanisms (supportive psychotherapy), looking at personality issues and conflicts (exploratory psychotherapy), changing thought processes (cognitive psychotherapy), or providing stress management and relaxation exercises (behavior therapy). Therapy may include combinations of the above, as well.

Other therapy options involve couples or family work. Talking things out with your partner or family members in the presence of a trained facilitator can be very helpful. Old tensions may worsen or new questions may arise. What should you tell your children? Who is going to cook when you are feeling ill?

Flexibility is the key in counseling; your therapy issues and needs may be very different at different points in your illness. At times you may not feel well enough to talk; other times you may wish to meet more frequently. A rigid therapist who is only willing to work in a set format is not going to be useful to you. Cancer is a roller-coaster ride; pick those who ride with you carefully.

Support Groups

Cancer support groups are becoming increasingly popular. It's no wonder; who better to talk to about cancer than others facing the same challenge? At the deepest level, the only people who understand what having cancer is like are others with cancer.

Just as with individual therapy, there are different kinds of support groups. Groups may be for people with cancer, family members, or both together. They may be for people with a specific type or stage of cancer, or for people undergoing a specific type of treatment. Groups may be time-limited (meet for certain duration, such as eight or ten sessions) or they may be ongoing, with no set ending date. They may meet weekly, every other week, or monthly. They may or may not be led by a professional. They may focus on supportive sharing, teaching by invited guests, visualization and relaxation exercises, or a combination of these formats.

To find the best group for you, start with your health care team. Groups may be offered on-site, or referrals can be given to local groups. Other sources of information on cancer support groups are your local American Cancer Society and Cancer Information Service (1-800-4-CANCER).

A support group may not immediately feel helpful. It is often difficult to hear about the hard times of others, and it may be difficult to share your feelings in front of strangers. You may get annoyed at or dislike other group members. After all, all kinds of people get cancer. Give yourself time to get used to the group and to the people. I recommend attending four to six sessions before deciding to leave a group. After that, it is possible that the group simply is not a good fit for your needs, or even that groups are not for you. As with everything else, trust your intuition and feelings; proceed on the course that feels best for you. For many, this path includes a support group of others with cancer.

Religion and Spirituality

Religion and spirituality can be powerful tools for coping with illness. This may involve traditional religious structure and institutions or your own individual beliefs and practices. Either way, this can be a profound source of comfort and understanding. Spiritual and religious views serve as a guidepost and anchor in times of stress and difficulty. At a time when you feel overwhelmed, religious and spiritual ideas help give an understanding of the unknown and a sense of the meaning of life and death. Spiritual traditions can provide a feeling of the world being much larger that your own individual problems. In addition, they offer an understanding of the purpose of your life as an individual human being.

Religious institutions also provide a sense of community. This helps you feel less alone as you face your illness. Considerable practical help is available, such as meals, transportation, and childcare. Certainly your openness to religion depends on your background and past experiences. Still, many have used cancer as an opportunity to begin exploration of spiritual issues. Many hospitals have chaplaincy services with personnel experienced in dealing with cancer-related issues.

Other Complementary Therapies

Mind/body approaches are numerous and are known by many names, including alternative, holistic, and unconventional. Here the term *complementary therapies* is used. This stresses the fact that they can be used *along with* conventional medical therapy, instead of in its place.

Physical approaches include exercise, yoga, massage, acupuncture, tai chi, chi gong, and other forms of bodywork. These are wonderful for keeping your body physically active. There is a lot that Western medicine does not understand about how the body works as a whole. The Eastern theory is that the body has channels of energy or life force (*chi*) that are opened and redirected through these various techniques. Many have been used for thousands of years.

Psychological methods include relaxation, visualization, meditation, hypnosis, counseling, and support groups. Relaxation, visualization, meditation, and hypnosis are all techniques to quiet and focus the mind. The benefits include an increased awareness and appreciation of the present moment and a feeling of connection and unity with other people and the world around you. Several of these techniques are described in Chapter 13, "Relaxation and Stress Reduction."

Spiritual avenues include prayer and spiritual counseling. Prayer, both by and for you, is getting a lot of attention these days. Some studies say it helps. It certainly can't hurt.

Creative Arts therapies include art, dance, drama, music, and writing therapies. Whether you are a beginner or expert in one or more of these techniques, a creative outlet for dealing with your feelings can be quite illuminating and useful. For many, feelings emerge more easily via a creative outlet than in traditional talking therapies.

I worked with a woman with breast cancer who struggled with the issue of complementary therapies. Friends and family members told her to meditate, visualize, and get acupuncture. Many of her friends said they had heard stories of "miracle cures" and urged her to try anything, including going to Mexico to try an untested medical treatment. She carefully talked through her options and decided against going to Mexico. Her family and friends were here, and she had developed a trusting relationship with her oncologist. Over time she decided to try a class on mindfulness meditation and found that it helped her feel relaxed and at peace with herself. She realized that it was not necessarily a cure for her cancer, but simply feeling better felt like an important and attainable goal. She remains in remission and is working and spending time with her family. She knows the future is uncertain, but says she feels she is learning to be more comfortable living with that uncertainty. After all, she says, the future is uncertain for everyone, even those without cancer.

Finding Your Own Path

Even with the support of your family, friends, and health care team, your cancer is a very personal and individual experience. It is a challenge to find your own way to treat and to live with illness. Have faith in your feelings, your hunches, and your intuitions. There is a fine balance to strive for, the balance between hope and acceptance. Hope for the best, hope for a cure, hope for the highest quality of life possible. At the same time, accept that there are no guarantees. Unfortunately, modern medicine does not have all the answers. Working with the system and accepting its limitations (as well as your own) is not easy, but it is crucial for your sense of well-being.

There Is No One Right Way

If there were one answer to cancer, everyone would follow the same recipe. Since there is not, there are confusing choices to be made. Gather all of the support and information that you feel you need. Discuss your choices with your physician and nurse. If certain complementary therapies feel right to you, do them. If not, don't. Be easy on yourself. Sometimes, after a diagnosis of cancer, people expect to change their personalities overnight. Eventually changes may occur, but, at least at the beginning, it is best to use the coping mechanisms that have helped you get through other difficulties in your life. You may be a person who copes with adversity by researching every bit of information available. If so, dive into the scientific literature. On the other hand, you may be a person who handles difficult situations by pulling back and allowing others to make decisions. Either way, do what works for you.

Individual Coping Styles

Many people will have their own ideas about what you should do and how you should feel. Some will want you to keep a stiff upper lip; others will urge you to let it all hang out. The bottom line is that no matter how things are physically, you are still you inside. People have different ways of coping. Some like to read every study on cancer; others leave that up to the doctor. Some meditate, do yoga, and acupuncture; others watch a movie, listen to music, pray, or work. Be yourself. Look back at the things (and the people) that have helped you get through hard times in the past. Life is full of challenges, and this includes unfairness and illness. As with other challenges, you will do the best you can.

Laughing and Loving

Laughter may not come easily, but when it does, let it happen. There is some evidence for the physiological benefits of laughter. It certainly can feel good. Humor involves looking at life from a different perspective. Often this can mean taking serious topics such as illness, life, and death and making fun of them in some way. I have had the good fortune of being witness to humor and mirth in some very unlikely and potentially uncomfortable situations. There is no better tension reliever. While not always an appropriate option, look for it when it is available.

Similarly, feelings of love and contentment may be difficult to find in a mind that is filled with lots of other details. Finding the time and space to live and love in a busy, imperfect, anxiety-filled world is a challenge faced by us all. We are all searching for meaning in our lives and our experiences. Sometimes meaning and peace are hidden behind what seems to be an insurmountable wall. The way through is not apparent. On second look, though, you may see gaps in the wall, tools to help you break through, or a way around.

One Day at a Time

The only moment any of us are living in is right now. Yesterday is gone; tomorrow may never come. This reality is never clearer than when you are dealing with a serious physical illness. Many have said that they never felt truly alive until they knew, at the deepest level, that they were going to die. Again, the operative word here is *challenge*. The challenge is to exist fully and love fully in the series of moments that go together to form today. In this way, the truly important things, your real priorities, show themselves to you.

This, of course, is much easier said than done. To live fully, one day at a time, when you are facing a difficult illness, is certainly not easy. To do it, treat your mind and body well. I wish you all the best on your journey.

About the Author

Burton A. Presberg, M.D., is Director of Psychosocial Services at the Alta Bates Comprehensive Cancer Center in Berkeley, California. He works closely with patients, families, and health care practitioners in addressing the multitude of biological, psychological, social, and spiritual issues involved in cancer.

Burt received his B.A. and M.D. degrees and psychiatric training from Cornell University. He received fellowship training in Consultation/Liasion Psychiatry and served on the faculty of the Medical College of Virginia in Richmond, Virginia prior to beginning his current position.

Suggested Reading

The volume of available literature is enormous and can be overwhelming. In keeping with the tone of the chapter, if it feels useful, read it; if not, put it away. Here are my suggestions of a few books that many have found helpful:

The Alpha Institute. 1993. *The Alpha Book on Cancer and Living*. A balanced, well researched, team-written book covering general cancer issues, conventional and alternative treatments, and coping.

Gordon, James S. 1996. *Manifesto For a New Medicine: Your Guide to Healing Partnerships and the Wise Use of Alternative Therapies.* Reading, Mass: Addison Wesley. An expert in alternative medicine describes a new model for modern medicine.

Jampolsky, Jerry. 1983. *Teach Only Love.* New York: Bantam Books. Written by the founder of the Center for Attitudinal Healing, this book offers an inspirational approach to love, acceptance, and healing.

Kabat-Zinn, John. 1994. *Wherever You Go, There You Are.* New York: Hyperian. Beautifully written essays on meditation, stress, and living in the moment. Not specifically focused on cancer.

Kushner, Harold S. 1981. *When Bad Things Happen to Good People.* New York: Avon Books. Written by a prominent clergyman struggling to come to terms with his son's illness and death.

Lasater, Judith. 1995. *Relax and Renew: Restful Yoga for Stressful Times.* Berkeley: Rodmell Press. Presents detailed step-by-step instructions and photographs of restorative yoga techniques.

Lerner, Michael. 1994. *Choices in Healing: Integrating the Best of Conventional and Complementary Approaches to Cancer.* Cambridge, Mass.: The MIT Press. Excellent, balanced review of complementary therapies by the founder of Commonweal.

Weil, Andrew. 1983. *Health and Healing.* Boston: Houghton-Mifflin. A leader in integrative medicine discusses his view of healing. One of a number of excellent books by Dr. Weil.

Wilber, Ken. 1991. *Grace and Grit.* Boston: Shambhala. Transpersonal psychologist Wilber and wife Treya's poignantly written account of Treya's breast cancer. Addresses questions about conventional and alternative medicine.

Http://www.salick.com A good place to start your search for cancer information on the Internet. Click on the "Resource Center" icon to begin. Be sure to check out Dr. Presberg's column "Mind and Body."

13

Relaxation and Stress Reduction

When you're faced with a threat, your body tenses and makes adrenaline. his stress response is designed to help you survive danger; it's a warning for you to flee or fight. But when stress becomes chronic, it dampens your immune system and makes it harder for your body to heal.

It's important while receiving cancer-fighting therapies to do everything in your power to keep your immune system strong. Relaxation techniques can not only help you feel less overwhelmed, but also help you reduce the immunity-suppressing effects of stress. Breathing, muscle relaxation, and imagery techniques, as well as self-hypnosis, can assist you in relaxing your body. Other techniques such as thought stopping and systematic desensitization can help you deal with specific fears.

Deep Breathing

Deep breathing is an ancient Eastern technique as well as a modern, medically proven adjunct to Western medicine. It oxygenates your blood while releasing muscle tension in your diaphragm. Deep breathing is an excellent way to achieve very rapid relaxation. It will help you feel better in a hurry when you're facing some immediate stress.

If you want to practice deep breathing, try lying down in a comfortable place. Bend your knees and lay one hand on your abdomen and the other on your chest. Breathe lightly through your nose. In this normal breathing pattern, the hand on your chest and the hand on your abdomen will rise and fall together. But in deep breathing, only the hand on your abdomen will rise, while your chest will move very slightly, if at all. By pushing your breath way down into your abdomen, you not only get more air, but you also stretch your diaphragm so that the tense abdominal muscles can start to relax.

Now try it. Breathe deeply so that only the hand on your abdomen rises with the breath. Breathe in slowly through your nose, pushing up the hand, and then exhale through your mouth. Sometimes it feels good to make a whooshing noise as you let go of the breath.

When you feel ready, take another breath. Breathe only when you feel like it. You're taking in a lot more air than usual, so you'll breathe more slowly than usual. If you rush it and breathe faster than you need to, you're going to get too much oxygen, and you may feel a little dizzy. If that happens, just concentrate on slowing your breathing so that you take a breath *only when you need to.*

If you have trouble pushing up the hand on your abdomen and only the hand on your chest seems to move, then you need more practice. One thing you can do is push down with the hand on your abdomen. While you're pushing down on your abdomen, try to use a deep breath to push it back up.

Practice the deep-breathing technique until you feel comfortable with it and it feels easy, almost second nature. You should set aside three or four times during the day to work on your breathing. When you've mastered deep breathing while lying down, practice it sitting in a chair, feet flat on the floor, hands resting on your knees. You'll find the practice comes in handy, because deep breathing is an extremely effective way of dealing with the tension you may feel while having an IV started or having your blood drawn in the lab.

Autogenic Breathing

Autogenic breathing combines deep breathing with imagery for extremely effective stress relief. To learn autogenic breathing, start by lying down and doing deep breathing for two to three minutes. When you're in a comfortable rhythm and feeling more relaxed, visualize yourself lying on a warm, white beach. Feel the warmth from the sun caress your skin, radiate into your muscles, and finally your bones. Feel the soft, warm breeze touch your body.

Now imagine being covered with warm sand; the weight of the sand feels like a warm, protective hand on your body. Feel the heavy warmth penetrate deep into your muscles, relaxing and purifying your body. The warmth and the heaviness relax your body more and more deeply.

Now listen to the ebb and flow of your breath. Say to yourself, "warm" as your breath comes in, and then "heavy" as your breath goes out. Warm on the in-breath, heavy on the out-breath. Warm and heavy, warm and heavy. Really try to feel the warmth in your limbs as you say "warm" on the in-breath. Try to visualize the heavy sand holding your body safe and secure as you breathe out.

Stay on the beach as long as you want, letting the autogenic breathing relax and refresh your body. Practice the imagery until the warmth and heaviness are easy to feel. Practicing this technique at home can pay off later, and the imagery can help you to relax even during extended treatments.

Other Relaxation Imagery

Visualization is a lovely way to take a break, a vacation from stress. You can go anywhere in your mind, creating a retreat of exquisite peace and beauty. The following three "retreats" will give you an idea of the special places you can go without ever leaving your chair. With just a little practice, you can start designing your own retreat that has all the elements you need for deep relaxation.

Retreat 1

It's dark and cool as you begin the path leading upward toward the mountain. Early morning stars and the moon guide you along this trail beside a rushing stream. Slowly you climb, step by step, along the flowered path wet with morning dew. The sky lightens into a pale blue. You know this day will be warm. Cardinals, bluebirds, and wrens start to whistle and sing, keeping you company along the path that begins to open into stands of pine and oak. You walk on, feeling strong and happy that you are alive and eager to stand atop the mountain at sunrise. The stream next to the path trickles over a tiny falls. You place your hand under it, drinking its clear, cold water. You walk on. Your body feels light and strong as you climb. The first golden rays of sunlight are just peeking out to your left as the trail reaches the edge of a granite knoll. You're at the top now, and the sun breaks behind the mountain range on the horizon, rising quickly, an enormous ball of power greeting you, warming you, lighting you. You sit on a rock, breathe deeply, inhale the clean, crisp air. In the valley below, you can see rivers of mist flowing. But here the warm, bright sun shines above you, strengthening you as it does the plants and the birds. Here at the top, you feel a sense of peace and relaxation flowing throughout your entire body.

Retreat 2

You awake slowly in your room by the ocean. Darkness envelopes you as you put on your beach slippers and pad out to the screen porch, warm cup in hand. You sit in the rocker, quietly rocking back and forth, listening to the roar of the cresting sea. The stars pierce the sky's black blanket. You breathe quietly, deeply, feeling the rolling of the rocker on the wooden floor. Near the shore, long grasses wave gently, mocking the movement of the sea. You are safe. The moist air caresses your face. The warm drink soothes. The sky lightens, and the stars disappear. You can see for miles. The sun rises red over the horizon as pelicans glide between the troughs of the soft sea swells. Light glows, bathing you. You continue to breathe deeply, slowly, mirroring the rhythm of the waves as they run up the shore.

Retreat 3

The weeks have been hectic, but you are safe now on the train. You sink deeply into your seat and watch the vast, pale desert slip past the train window. Buttes stand silent and orange above the sagebrush-covered ground. The sun is setting, and the sky flames red and purple. The light fades slowly, but you can still see the mountains cut against the night sky. The low, rocking thunder of the train wheels blankets all other sounds. You feel safe and peaceful as the train rocks gently under you. You sink more deeply into your seat as you hear the clacking wheels. You have no problems to solve, nothing to think about as the train carries you through the desert night. It holds you, rocking gently as it speeds.

Your retreat may be nothing like these. You may call up a room from childhood, the breakfast table at your grandmother's house, a Paris cafe, a sandbar at the bend of a river, a high meadow, a campground beneath whispering trees. Go there often; use your retreat when you feel anxious and tired, when you are uncomfortable, when you are bored.

Imagery and Healing

Imagery is a powerful tool that can do far more than relax you. Imagery can also help you to heal. O. Carl Symonton, in his book *Getting Well Again*, shows how certain kinds of imagery may increase your ability to fight cancer. Symonton encourages people to imagine ferocious white blood cells tearing and consuming the weak cancer cells. Or you can visualize the chemotherapy as a powerful chemical that surrounds and destroys cancer cells. Symonton believes that *how* you visualize the cancer, the chemotherapy, and the white cells is very important. Read his book to learn more about how his use of visualization can help you.

While Symonton's techniques are widely used, there are many other approaches to healing visualizations. Many people use images of white light that soothes and heals a specific body area. Samples of healing visualizations can be found in *Visualization for Change* by Patrick Fanning. A sample script and instructions for making your own visualization tape are included in Chapter 14.

Progressive Muscle Relaxation

Progressive muscle relaxation (PMR) is a technique developed in the 1920s by Dr. Edmund Jacobson. It is based on the theory that a person cannot be both relaxed and anxious at the same time.

To calm anxiety, muscles are progressively tightened and released in sequence throughout your entire body.

In the beginning, PMR takes fifteen to twenty minutes for each practice session. But in a few weeks, after you learn it thoroughly, you can tighten groups of muscles simultaneously and reduce the time spent to just a few minutes. When using this technique, avoid tensing muscles or areas of your body that may be painful. If pain is a problem, just read this section to learn the PMR sequences, and then go on to the next section, "Relaxation without Tension," to use this technique in a safer way.

Basic PMR Procedure

First, tighten your right fist and forearm. Clench as hard as you can for seven seconds. Notice what the tension feels like. Now release your fist and feel the muscles in your forearm relax for twenty seconds. Notice how relaxation feels—heavy, warm, or tingly. Really experience the relaxation in your hand and forearm. Repeat the procedure with your right fist once again, always noticing as you relax the release of the tension. Now do the same thing with your left fist and forearm. Tense for seven seconds and relax for twenty. Now do both fists at the same time, tensing for seven seconds and relaxing for twenty. Always notice how relaxation feels in your muscles.

The next step is to tense the muscles in your right arm. Make them as hard as you can for seven seconds and then relax. Do the tensing and relaxing twice with each arm.

As you continue through the exercise, tighten each specific muscle for seven seconds and relax for twenty. And then repeat the same muscle once again. Pay attention to what relaxation feels like in each muscle.

Now focus on your face, the seat of so much tension. Wrinkle up your forehead. Hold it taut, then release.

Now frown and squint your eyes, holding them tightly shut. Release.

Purse your mouth into an "O." Relax and notice what it's like to let go of tension in this area of your face.

Now tighten your jaw, bite hard, and push your tongue against the roof of your mouth. Relax and notice what it feels like to release the tension in your jaw.

Turning to the neck and shoulder area, press your head back against your chair and then relax your head. Roll slowly and gently to the right and then to the left.

Straighten your head and gently let it fall forward. Relax and really feel the release of tension in your neck.

Now hunch your shoulders. Relax and let them droop, feeling the relaxation spread through your neck, throat, and shoulders.

Feel the relaxation move throughout your entire body. Feel the comfort of the heaviness. Now breathe in and fill your lungs completely. Hold your breath and notice the tension. As you exhale, feel all tension leaving your body. Repeat the full breath several times, paying attention to how tension can drain out of your body as you exhale.

Tighten your abdominal muscles, just as if you were preparing to be punched. When you relax, let the tension drain away again. Put your hand on your belly and push it up with a deep breath. As you let go, feel your entire abdomen relax.

Gently arch your back slightly. Be careful not to strain it. Relax again and take another deep breath.

Tighten the muscles in your lower back. Relax and notice how the muscles feel without tension.

Tighten your buttocks and thighs. Flex your thighs by pressing down your heels as hard as you can. Relax and notice what it's like to let go of tension in these big muscles.

Now curl your toes downward, making your calves tense. Relax.

Now pull your toes back toward your face, creating tension in your shins. Relax again. Observe the muscles in your feet and calves. Notice how it feels for them finally to relax.

Just feel the heaviness throughout your lower body as relaxation deepens. Notice the relaxation in your feet, ankles, calves, shins, knees, thighs, and buttocks. Let the relaxation spread to your stomach, lower back, and chest. Let it become deeper and deeper. Experience the relaxation deepening in your shoulders, neck, arms, and hands. Then experience the feeling of looseness and relaxation in your neck, jaw, and all your facial muscles. Your whole body feels more and more deeply relaxed.

Shorthand PMR Procedure

After you've practiced PMR for several weeks and are aware of the effects of tension and relaxation on specific muscles, you're ready to shorten the process. You can now tighten and relax certain muscle groups simultaneously. Just as you did before, tighten for seven seconds and relax for twenty, but be sure to avoid painful areas or straining. Carefully observe the effects of both the contraction and the relaxation of your muscles. As your muscles loosen, let your whole body grow heavy and still.

1. Curl your fists. Tighten your biceps and forearms (in a "Charles Atlas" pose). Relax.

2. Wrinkle your forehead. At the same time, press your head as far back as possible, rolling it clockwise in a complete circle. Reverse the direction of the roll. Now wrinkle up the muscles of your face like a walnut. Frown with your eyes squinted, lips pursed, tongue pressed against the roof of your mouth. And with the same walnut face, hunch your shoulders. Relax.

3. Breathe deeply into your abdomen as you slightly arch your back. Hold, observe, and relax. Breathe deeply again, pressing out your abdomen. Hold. And then relax.

4. Now curl your toes while simultaneously tightening your calves, thighs, and buttocks. Relax. Pull your feet and toes back toward your face, tightening your shins. Hold and relax.

Relaxation without Tension

This exercise involves relaxing your muscles in the same sequence that you learned with PMR. But there's one difference: you don't tighten each muscle. Instead, you notice any tension that may exist in the muscle and then "relax away" the tightness.

Twice a day practice going though each muscle in the PMR sequence and "relaxing away" any tension you find. Try to make the muscle feel as relaxed as it did right after you let go in the PMR exercise.

Relaxation without tension allows you to scan your body for "hot spots" of tightness. There's no embarrassing process that others might observe. You can relax away tension in the doctor's office or the clinic. You can use this technique to relax away tension while you're receiving treatments.

Self-Hypnosis

This is an extremely effective technique for relaxing your body and strengthening your mind. You can use hypnosis to seed affirmations and positive thoughts that will help you get through having blood tests, chemotherapy, radiation, and other treatment procedures. Self-hypnosis makes you relax in the moment. Through the power of suggestion, it also helps you relax long after the trance state has ended. When you suggest to yourself during hypnosis that you'll feel more calm or confident during a particularly stressful procedure, the chances are that you really will feel that way. Here's how you do it.

To induce hypnosis, plan for a twenty-minute session. Loosen your clothing and lie or sit in a comfortable place. Select words such as "relax" or "peaceful and strong" that you can repeat mentally during the induction. These will be cue words that help you to deepen your level of relaxation. Before starting the induction, you should also choose an affirmation or suggestion for your subconscious to carry into the future when you're facing stressful procedures (see the list of affirmations later in this chapter for suggestions).

Close your eyes and feel your eyelids begin to get heavy. Take a deep breath, way down into your abdomen. And as you exhale, feel the relaxation spread throughout your entire body. Take another deep breath, and as you exhale say to yourself your cue word or phrase that will deepen the relaxation.

Now begin to focus on your legs. Imagine that they have become heavy lead weights. Tell yourself that your legs are becoming heavier and heavier, more and more deeply relaxed. Just repeat the phrases: "Heavier and heavier, heavy and letting go, heavy and relaxed, more and more deeply relaxed."

When you achieve a sense of heaviness in your legs, turn your attention to your arms. Your arms, too, can become heavier and heavier, heavy and relaxed, becoming more and more deeply relaxed as you feel them letting go. Just repeat these phrases in any combination until your arms truly begin to feel heavy. Then repeat the same phrases for both your arms and your legs.

Now turn your attention to your face. Suggest to yourself that your forehead is becoming as smooth as silk, smooth and relaxed. Your cheeks, too, are smooth and relaxed. Your forehead and cheeks are more and more deeply relaxed, letting go of tension, feeling smooth and relaxed. Repeat these phrases until you feel that your face has let go of all muscular tension.

Now focus on your jaw. Suggest that your jaw is becoming loose and relaxed. Suggest that as your jaw becomes more and more deeply relaxed, you'll feel the muscles letting go and your lips beginning to part. Repeat the phrase "loose and relaxed" until you feel your jaw let go of tension.

Now turn your attention to your neck and shoulders. Suggest that your neck is centered and relaxed. Your shoulders are relaxed and drooping. Take a slow breath and let the relaxation deepen in your neck and shoulders.

Take another deep breath, and as you exhale let the relaxation spread into your chest, stomach, and back. Take several more deep breaths. As you exhale, let the feelings of relaxation deepen in your torso.

Now it's time to go to a special place. A place of safety and peace. It may be at the beach or on a mountaintop or maybe a room from your childhood. It may be a place where you always felt loved and accepted. Your special place can be a real location or something entirely made up. In a moment you'll walk there. You can imagine reaching your special place by descending a flight of stairs or walking down a forest path or entering a gate. In ten steps you'll be there. With each step you'll grow more and more deeply relaxed, feeling peaceful and safe as you move toward your special place.

Now you will grow more relaxed with each step: ten . . . nine . . . eight . . . seven . . . six . . . five . . . four . . . three . . . two . . . one . . . zero. (If you want to go through the countdown two or even three times to deepen hypnosis, that's perfectly fine.)

In your special place, you can further deepen the feelings of relaxation. The following suggestions can be made in any order. Repeat them over and over again, until you reach a state of deep calm.

Drifting deeper and deeper, deeper, and deeper.

More and more drowsy, peaceful, and calm.

Drifting and drowsy, drowsy, and drifting.

Drifting down, down, down into total relaxation.

After you've given yourself these deepening suggestions, let yourself relax and enjoy your special place. Now is a good time to repeat the suggestion or affirmation that you've prepared before hypnosis. Suggestions that others have used include affirmations like these:

I am feeling stronger each day.

I can relax during the chemotherapy/radiation therapy.

The treatments will make me healthier and healthier.

The cancer is dying; the treatments are killing it.

I feel strengthened by the love of my friends and family.

I can relax and let the chemotherapy/radiation work.

Once you've repeated your suggestion or affirmation several times, you can bring yourself up to normal consciousness any time you wish. To come all the way up, simply count from one to ten. After you get to around five, suggest to yourself that you're getting more and more alert, refreshed, and wide awake. Keep making these suggestions as you count the remaining numbers and begin opening your eyes around the count of nine.

Don't try to drive or do anything that requires focused attention immediately after hypnosis. Relax for a little while longer and enjoy the feelings of calm that hypnosis usually brings.

Thought Stopping

When someone says, "Cancer treatments make me nervous," this statement makes sense intuitively. But it isn't really true. It isn't chemotherapy or radiation therapy that makes people nervous. Rather, the anxiety results from a series of *thoughts* and *worries* about the treatments. If you can pay attention to what you say to yourself about the things that scare you, you will see how your thoughts can add to your anxiety. Here is a list of some of the things that one man thought just before treatment:

How many times will they have to stick me today before they get the IV right?

I wonder how sick I'll feel?

I hate the whole procedure, I hate sitting here.

What if I feel really weak?

I wonder if I'm going to be able to keep working.

These drugs are too strong; maybe they'll do more harm than good.

These thoughts, and a host of others like them, had made him nervous. Each frightening thought triggered the production of adrenaline, which only increased his feelings of anxiety and set off another round of scary thoughts. This process is known as the *anxiety feedback loop*: thoughts anticipating danger or pain cause the body to produce adrenaline. The adrenaline, in turn, stimulates the lymbic area of your brain so that you feel anxious.

The anxiety seems to confirm your sense of danger, which then stimulates more thoughts of pain and catastrophe. The feedback loop can keep your anxiety spiraling upward till you feel tremendously upset.

Breaking the Loop

Thought stopping is an important technique for interrupting the feedback loop. If you shut off the frightening thoughts and the adrenaline surge that each thought triggers, you can start to calm down.

Here's how it works. Whenever you feel anxious, check to see what you're thinking. Notice if you're anticipating pain or problems—anything that's scary. Then shout "Stop!" to yourself. Just really scream it internally. You need to make the "Stop!" loud so that you can interrupt the flow of fear-provoking thoughts. If you can't interrupt the thoughts by commanding them to stop, you'll need something more imperative. Clap your hands or shout out loud (if no one's around to hear you). Or snap a rubber band around your wrist—the sharp sting will help to break the chain of thoughts.

Stop and Breathe

Once you've stopped the thoughts, you'll need something to replace them. Nature hates a vacuum; the negative thoughts will soon return if nothing fills the gap. You've already learned deep breathing. As soon as you interrupt the flow of thoughts, start taking slow, deep breaths. Really try to stretch and relax your diaphragm. Focus all your attention on your breathing, feeling its warmth permeate your body.

Now count your breaths. On each exhalation count, "One . . . two . . . three . . . four." After your fourth exhalation, start over again with one. Focus on the counting until your inner talk falls still, your anxiety lessens, and your mind becomes peaceful.

After you finish counting your breaths, don't worry if negative thoughts come back again. They frequently do. Immediately counter them by shouting "Stop!" and beginning to focus on your breathing. Count your breaths for one or two minutes and see if you're feeling calmer. Some people have to stop anxious thoughts over and over again as they anticipate a stressful situation. That's okay. The important thing is not to let the anxious thoughts take root, not to dwell on them. Each anxious thought you stop protects you from a burst of adrenaline and a subsequent increase in your nervousness. This is hard work, but it pays off big dividends by lowering your overall stress level.

Affirmations

In addition to counting your breaths, you can replace frightening thoughts with positive affirmations. An affirmation is a short, pithy statement that helps you feel more self-confident, stronger, and less fearful.

Here is a list of affirmations that you may use. Choose a few that you like and memorize them. Or use them for ideas to create unique affirmations of your own.

About Relaxation

- Relaxation floods my body like a healing golden light.
- Each breath brings a flood of healing power to every corner of my body.
- I am filled with peace, calm, and serenity.
- Relaxation, enjoyment, and love are the things that keep me well.
- Taking care of myself keeps me strong.
- Relaxation is the gift I give myself.
- Every time I breathe in, I bring a wave of peace and relaxation. Every time I breathe out, I let go of tension and fear.

To Reduce Fear about Treatments

- I can get through this.
- I can take care of myself.
- I can ask for what I need.
- The people around me (my nurse, my doctor, my family) know how to make sure that I am safe and comfortable.
- Every treatment takes me another step closer towards health and recovery.
- Cancer cells are weak, sick, and confused.

- Chemotherapy/radiation therapy is a strong ally. It works with my body's natural defenses to wipe out the defective cancer cells.

- I am open to the healing power of the medications/radiation.

After Chemotherapy or Radiation Therapy Treatments

- The chemotherapy has done its job. Now it will be washed out of my body, taking with it the dead cancer cells.

- My body's natural defenses are building again and will be ready to protect me again.

- Chemotherapy/radiation therapy is like a great crashing wave. It may shake me up for a minute, but now the water has receded, and I am safe again on the shore.

- Chemotherapy/radiation therapy is like a torrential downpour, washing away the weak and broken cancer cells, leaving the strong healthy cells glistening in the sun.

- Chemotherapy/radiation therapy has been like allied troops coming to a troubled area, routing the enemy, then returning the region to peace and beauty and health.

Systematic Desensitization

Some people are tremendously afraid of needles; some fear the symptoms or sensations surrounding chemotherapy or radiation therapy. If you have strong fears about the treatments, deep breathing and muscle relaxation may not be enough to achieve calm. Fortunately, there is a highly effective method for dealing with strong fears that you can use on your own or with the help of a counselor. *Systematic desensitization* was developed in the 1950s by Joseph Wolpe and has had an excellent forty-five-year track record of helping people overcome fear.

Systematic desensitization allows you to imagine scenes of higher and higher levels of anxiety while maintaining complete physical relaxation. You move incrementally, scene by scene, from the least anxiety-evoking to the most stressful situation you can imagine. One emotion (relaxed calm) is used to counteract another (anxiety). Even the most threatening situations can be gotten used to—if you do it gradually, step by step.

Here's what you do. Everything in systematic desensitization depends on constructing an appropriate *hierarchy*. This is a list of stressful situations that ranges from almost no anxiety to the highest level of fear. For instance, to construct your hierarchy, imagine having to deal with the chemotherapy or radiation therapy experience. Think first about the least threatening part of it, perhaps imagining yourself removed in space or time from the whole situation. Low-stress items on your hierarchy might include dressing to go to the clinic or even making an appointment for your chemotherapy or radiation therapy treatments. Items that are more anxiety-evoking would place you closer in time or space to the experience. For you, these experiences might include checking in with the receptionist at the clinic or having the nurse wipe your arm with alcohol before inserting the IV or changing into a gown and lying on the radiation table. Items at the top end of the hierarchy would be the part of the experience you fear most. This might be the needle stick, the sensation of the drug entering your veins, being positioned on the radiation table, or a particular side effect.

Go ahead now and try to develop your own scenes for a hierarchy. You need between eight and twenty scenes. Some people like to write the scenes down randomly, just as they come to mind. Others put the least scary scene at the top of a piece of paper and the most frightening one at the bottom. Then they try to fill in six or more scenes of graduated intensity in between. However you do it, when you've finally thought of enough scenes for an eight- to twenty-item hierarchy, put them in order down a page from the least to most stressful.

Here's a sample hierarchy from a 43-year-old woman who was facing her third chemotherapy treatment. A similar hierarchy can be constructed to help lessen anxiety about radiation therapy.

1. Thinking about going for treatment.

2. Preparing for treatment—shopping and preparing meals in advance, arranging childcare, arranging my work schedule.

3. Going to the lab for blood tests two days before chemotherapy.

4. Waking up on the morning of the day of the treatment.

5. Riding to the clinic.

6. Checking in with the receptionist.

    7. Sitting in the waiting room.

    8. Waiting for the doctor.

    9. Waiting in the treatment area for my turn.

  10. Watching the nurse prepare the IV bags, tubing, and syringes.

  11. Preparing to have the IV started—the feel of the tourniquet, the smell of alcohol.

  12. Having the needle inserted and feeling the medicine going into my veins.

Notice that each item on the hierarchy is a little more stressful than the one before it. The important thing is to make the hierarchy *graduated* so that there is only a small increase in anxiety level from item to item.

Desensitization Procedure

Once you've developed your hierarchy, it's time to start using it. Here's what you do.

    1. Relax. Start each desensitization session by taking ten to fifteen minutes to relax. Use deep breathing and progressive muscle relaxation to make your body as free of stress as possible.

    2. Visualize a peaceful scene. Use the special place that you imagined while practicing hypnosis or think of a place where you feel safe, calm, and peaceful. It could be in the mountains or the beach, real or imagined, indoors or outdoors. It doesn't matter as long as you can vividly create the image. Practice visualizing the scene right now. See the shapes and colors, hear the sounds, feel the texture, the temperature. Make the scene and feelings as real and detailed as possible.

    3. Start the first scene of your hierarchy. After you feel really relaxed, switch from your peaceful place to the first scene of your hierarchy. This scene, too, should be as vivid as possible. Create as much detail as you can so that it feels as if you're right there. Don't picture yourself feeling any particular emotion; just imagine the situation. Should you feel any anxiety, stop the image immediately and return to your peaceful place. If you don't feel anxiety, continue to visualize this first item from your hierarchy for thirty seconds. When you can visualize a scene twice without anxiety, go on to the next item on your hierarchy.

4. **What to do between scenes.** When you've stopped visualizing a scene from your hierarchy—either because you feel anxious or you've visualized it for the full thirty seconds—take a deep breath and return to your peaceful scene. Do the relaxation-without-tension exercise described earlier in this chapter. Focus on each of your muscle groups in sequence, relaxing away any tension that you find. When you feel calm and relaxed, go back to your hierarchy.

5. **Progress through your hierarchy.** Never stay in a scene that makes you anxious. Cut it off immediately and return to the peaceful place. If one scene continues to make you anxious time after time, skip it and work it in farther up your hierarchy. It's probably more anxiety-provoking than you thought and belongs up with the more stressful items. Make your first desensitization session no more than fifteen or twenty minutes. Later sessions can be stretched to as much as half an hour. Expect to master no more than two or three scenes in each session. If you find that your anxiety is high for every scene, it probably means that you need to relax more deeply—both at the onset and during the interval between hierarchy scenes. If you put more time into the relaxation process, you may find that you desensitize more quickly to the frightening images.

6. **When you finish.** When you complete your hierarchy, expect your anxiety to be improved but not absent. Cancer-fighting treatments may no longer be overwhelming, but they won't be a walk in the park either. The important thing is that you *can* reduce your anxiety. You can reduce it to a point where you're able to cope and get through the experience.

14

Scripts for Relaxation and Visualization Tapes

Body Relaxed—Mind at Ease
Peaceful Body, Quiet Mind
by Harriet Sanders Karis, L.C.S.W.

How to Use the Scripts

To obtain maximum benefit from these four scripts, it is best to either have them recorded or read aloud by another person to you. In either case, the scripts should be narrated in a slow, soothing, relaxing tone, with ample time allowed for the formation of images and follow-through with other suggestions. When making your own tape, you may wish to use pleasant background music. Just make sure that any music you record does not overpower or compete with the narration.

The relaxation and visualization scripts given here are designed to be used together—the relaxation scripts provide the lead-ins to the two visualization scripts. They may, however, be used separately. When using the relaxation script alone, be sure to allow time at the end to come out of the relaxed state. You may want to include a modification of the last paragraph of the visualization script or other similar suggestions that would gradually lead you back into an awakened state.

Use the scripts as frequently as you like. The more you use them, the easier the process will become for you and undoubtedly the more beneficial the results will be. Using the script in the middle of the day can provide a refreshing break and at bedtime a delightful prelude to a restful night's sleep. Listening to the script before, during, or after treatment is highly recommended to offset stress, anxiety, or discomfort.

You may either sit in a chair or lie down when listening to the tape or having the script read to you. The ideal position is simply the one that works best for you. Feel free to experiment. Find a comfortable place to relax—one that is quiet and where you will not be disturbed. Dim the lights. Settle in and *enjoy!*

Relaxation Script 1

Body Relaxed—Mind at Ease

And now it is time to become still and relax. Time to turn within, to journey to that special place deep inside you that knows only peace; only comfort; only calm. Find a comfortable position in your chair. You may want to rest your hands gently in your lap or on your knees or let your arms just dangle at your sides. There is no right or wrong way to relax, just whatever feels right for you, and if you haven't already done so, you may want to gently close your eyes, letting the closing of your eyes be a signal to the outside world that, for this next little while, you are going to detach, to let go, to turn within. Let go all of tension and strain. This is not a time to be thinking about outer concerns, stresses, or worries. This is a time just to be still. Still your body now and quiet your thoughts. Throughout this entire exercise, know that you will always be in control—that there is nothing to fear. So let go now. Allow your mind and body to be at rest and gently release into the calm.

Focus now on your breathing. For the next few breaths, breathe in slowly and deeply through your nose and, at the top of the inhale, hold it—and now breathe out softly and slowly through your mouth. Once again breathe in slowly, through your nose—hold it—now breathe out, gradually and softly, through your mouth. As you exhale now, experience the flow of your breath as it gently and evenly exits your body; feel that wonderful sense of stillness and peace that comes as you release. Once more now, breathe in slowly through your nose—hold it—now breathe out, gradually and slowly, through your mouth. Breathe normally now, without effort, without strain—just let your body follow the natural rhythm, the natural cadence set by your breathing, and allow it to move you deeper and deeper into the calm. Should you find any outer thoughts attempting to intrude and compete with this state of peace that is engulfing you now, just let these thoughts gently pass through and then fade away into nothingness. Let them go. If you find yourself beginning to nod off to sleep, or if the sound of my voice trails in and trails out, that's okay. Whatever works for you will be just fine. So just relax and let go. Any outer noise, any outer distraction that you might hear will only serve to move you farther and farther away and deeper and deeper into the calm. Now focus again on your breathing, and this time, as you inhale, I want you to silently say to yourself the word *let*, and as you exhale silently, say the word *go*. Breathing in: *let*, breathing out: *go*. *Let go. Let go. Let go.* It is okay to let go. It is safe to let go. For it is in letting go of all outer stresses, all tension, all distress, and *dis-ease*—it is in the letting go of these experiences that you open to the healing your body so desperately needs for the restoration to health and wholeness. So fear not, resist not, just let go. All is well.

Now feel this relaxing sense of calm beginning to fill your body. I want you to imagine this beautiful sense of relaxation, imagine it being a white, puffy cloud of light that begins to ascend your body at your feet. Feel this beautiful cloud of light as it moves in and between your toes, allow it to travel along the soles of your feet, up into your heels and into your ankles. Just feel both your feet now immersed in this soft, billowy cloud of light. Feel all the tightness in your feet beginning now to dissipate, as your muscles relax and let go—leaving you with the feeling of your feet just merging into the floor. Feel this white, puffy cloud of light, this relaxing sense of calm, feel it now as it moves up into your legs. Let it move gradually along your shins and feel it as it softly massages and kneads the muscles there in your calves. Feel your legs becoming very limp and loose now as all the tension drains from them. Let go in your knee joints and in your thighs. As you let go in your thighs, just imagine this billowy cloud of light moving through your thighs, lulling all your muscles there to relax; softening them into a state of peace and calm. As you let go in your thighs, you might notice that your thighs begin to part a bit, and that's okay. Just imagine all the tension of the day, all concerns you may have, just feel all of this being drained away through your thighs and channeled out from your body. Focus now on your buttocks and, as you inhale, I want you to squeeze the muscles there in your buttocks—squeeze them tightly. Squeeze the muscles in your buttocks and your abdomen and pelvic area. Squeeze tightly now. As you exhale, release and gently let go. Just let it all hang loose and feel that wonderful sense of peace that comes as you release the tightness and allow the softness, the peace, the stillness to set in. Feel the sense of peace and comfort now in your abdominal area; that area that can hang onto so much tightness and so much tension. Feel the muscles in your abdomen now just soften and loosen and let go. Just imagine all the little organs there in your abdomen breathing a collective sigh of relief as all the tension just drains away, and they are left afloat in a sea of peaceful calm. Know that, as you deepen into this state of serenity and peace, all fear just dissipates; for fear and peace cannot coexist. As you relax, as you become still, you are at peace. Feel this white, puffy cloud of light, this relaxing sense of calm, feel it now, as it moves up into your chest area and, as you inhale now, just imagine you are drawing this beautiful cloud of light into your lungs. And, as you exhale, just let your entire rib cage softly fall, softly fall into this beautiful cloud of light. Notice now how much smoother, how much gentler your breathing is now. As you focus on your breathing once more, notice the peace and the tranquillity that there is now, as you breathe in and breathe out, breathe in and breathe out, breathe in and breathe out. Imagine this white, puffy cloud of light, this relaxing sense of calm, imagine it now flowing along your breast bone, feel it as it moves up into your shoulders now, soothing and smoothing away whatever pockets of tension might be stored there. And, as you relax in your shoulders, you might notice that your shoulders begin to droop a bit, and that's okay. Hold onto nothing. Hold onto nothing except this wonderful sense of relaxation and peace that you are experiencing now. Allow this relaxing sense of calm now to spill over into your upper back, that area that can hang onto so much tension and so much tightness. Feel the muscles there in your upper back now just give way to this sense of peace and feel all the tightness there begin to unfurl. Let all the tension just fade away. Imagine this beautiful cloud of light, this wonderful sense of calm, imagine it now, cascading all the way down your spinal column; and, as you release in your spine, imagine that your vertebrae, one by one, begin to sink deeper and deeper and deeper into the calm.

Now prepare for the last vestiges of tension to be removed from your upper body as you focus now on your arms and imagine this white, puffy cloud of light. Imagine it now as it floats down your upper arms; feel it as it flows into your elbows, down now into your forearms. Let it stream now into your wrists and flow ever so gently now into the palms of your hands, all the way out to the very tips of your fingers. Just feel your arms becoming so heavy now, as all the tension just fades away. You might notice now that your shoulders may even droop more now as you find it harder and harder to resist the pull to let go and relax. You might even notice that the tips of your fingers begin to tingle a bit as the last vestiges of tension drain through them.

You are doing so well now. Your body is responding perfectly. Continue now in this state, letting nothing distract you. Close the door on any unwanted thoughts. And any outside noises that you might hear will only serve to move you farther and farther away and deeper and deeper into this state of stillness and peace.

Feel this white, puffy cloud of light, this relaxing sense of calm, feel it as it moves up into your neck area, and allow the muscles there at the base of your head just to loosen and let go. You might notice that this causes your head to tilt forward a bit, and that's okay. Just let go. Feel this sense of stillness now, as it comes over your throat area. And just imagine your vocal cords at rest now, all movement around your throat stilled—silenced by this beautiful sense of calm. Let go in your jaw and, as you let go in your jaw, your lips might part a bit, and that's okay. Again, hold onto nothing. Feel this wonderful sense of peace now, as it permeates your mouth. Feel the quietness and the stillness settling in at the back of your throat. Notice how comfortable it is to have your tongue resting so quietly on the floor of your mouth or nestled against your upper palate. Feel this relaxing sense of calm, this white, puffy cloud of light, as it moves upward now into your face. Feel it as it begins to pulsate along your cheekbones, spanning out now, to touch that area around your temples and your ears. Imagine that you can feel yourself being gently massaged around your temples, encouraged to just let go. Feel all the tension draining now from your face, all traces of tightness or tautness just fading away. Feel this relaxing sense of calm, this white, puffy cloud of light, feel it now as it begins to move along the bridge of your nose, feel it now as it streams out now to touch the areas there around your eyes, and feel the muscles there, in the corners of your eyes, just loosen and let go and free themselves of any tightness you might have been carrying there. Relax the area in between your brow. As you loosen and free yourself of all traces of tension in your face, you might notice that your face becomes a bit warm, much as if you had your face turned to the rays of the sun and it was beaming softly down upon you. Feel this sense of calm now as it moves up into your forehead, soothing and smoothing away whatever tightness or tension you might be carrying there. Let this sensation comfort you, much as if a gentle hand was softly stroking your brow. And finally, allow this relaxing sense of calm, this white, puffy cloud of light, allow it now to move up into your scalp area, smoothing away whatever tightness or tension you might be carrying on the surface of your head. In your mind's eye now, just imagine this white, puffy cloud of light; imagine it seeping down into the very pores of your scalp. Allow it to infiltrate the innermost recesses of your mind, sweeping away whatever tension-filled thoughts or fear-filled emotions that might be stored there. And, as this beautiful sense of relaxation and calm flows unencumbered now, just imagine your entire mind being bathed in clarity and light and filled with images and thoughts of comfort, serenity and peace.

You are so relaxed now, from the top of your head, to the very tips of your toes. You are at peace. Calm in mind, calm in heart, calm in body.

Visualization Script 1

The Rainbow

You are so relaxed. Your whole being is so tranquil and still. It's as if someone has turned out all the lights in the house you call your body, and all your muscles, cells, and organs are fast asleep, nestled into a state of calm repose and rest. No matter what may be occurring on the outside, hold this image of your body being totally relaxed and at peace. Pay close attention to your breathing. Breathe slowly, in and out, through your nose. Breathe evenly, slowly, gently. Let your inhale come softly and then release gently into the exhale, without effort, force, or strain. Let no outer activity distract you; just become lost in the rhythmic flow of your breathing. Notice the feelings and sensations as air flows in and then flows out your body. And now, with each inhale, I want you to imagine that you are being softly swept up; and with each exhale, imagine that you are being gently pushed far, far, away. Feel yourself drifting now, being lifted up and carried away by the movement of your breathing. Inhale, and feel yourself being swept up. Exhale, and let yourself be pushed far, far away.

Now, in your mind's eye, allow yourself to be transported to a beautiful meadow. It has just rained, and the earth smells of fresh moisture. Breathe deeply and allow the smell of damp earth to penetrate your nostrils. It delights you! You look at the grass and the foliage of the trees and notice that they glisten with newly fallen raindrops—creating the illusion of tiny sunbeams all about you. Everything is so clean, so fresh, so pure. You look down at your feet and notice that nestled there among the glistening blades of grass is a most beautiful rainbow that extends outward from your feet in a small arc, curved like a horseshoe. One end of the rainbow connects with your right foot, and the other end with your left. As you gaze at this rainbow you cannot help but be amazed at how beautifully the colors harmonize and blend with each other. Colors of red, blue, orange, yellow, and green. You can even feel the vibrations of energy emanating from these colors as they softly connect with your feet.

And now let yourself focus on the red ray of the rainbow. It's the color nearest to you. And imagine that as you inhale you are drawing this ray of color in through your feet and up into your body. Feel the flow of the color red as it moves throughout your body like warm liquid light. The color red symbolizes life, strength, power, and vitality. Feel the movement of this color as it travels upward into your body—through your legs and thighs, your hips, your abdomen, your chest, your shoulders. Allow it to move along your back and through your arms. Picture it now as it moves into your neck and face and head. Envelope your body in the color red. Let it pulsate to this color—and as it does, experience your body becoming alive, vital, and strong. And as you feel yourself fully saturated with this red ray of light, let it flow from your body through the crown of your head and form an arch directly above you.

Now focus again on the rainbow at your feet. Inhale deeply and this time draw the color orange into your body. Let it flow into your lower body, upward into your abdomen, into your upper body until you are permeated throughout with the color orange. Orange symbolizes optimism, self-confidence, enthusiasm, and courage. Allow it to flow freely to those areas in your body where you are experiencing doubt or fear. Draw out the courage and optimism you can feel in this color. And now let this color emerge through the top of your head and join the color red in the arch above you.

And now draw in the yellow ray of the rainbow through your feet. Let it rise like warm liquid light and gently flow throughout your being. Yellow symbolizes mental or intellectual power, wisdom, happiness, and joy. Take delight now as you picture you entire body filled with the color yellow. Feel every organ and cell in your body opening to the uplifting, positive, joy-filled vibration of this color. Let this color stream into any areas of your body that are in pain or that ache with sadness. See these areas open like lotus petals to take in the soothing, warm, glowing rays of yellow light. See it infusing every atom, every cell of your body with the wisdom and understanding needed to restore your body to perfect health. And now allow the yellow color to exit your body and join the rays of red and orange arched above your head.

Look down at your feet now and see the green ray of the rainbow preparing to move into your body. Green symbolizes balance, peace, growth, and healing. Allow this color to enfold you, and feel it injecting your entire being with its healing and harmonizing power. As this color flows through your body now, visualize it sparking the growth of new and healthy cells—cells that will quickly outnumber and overpower the confused and unhealthy ones that are causing your illness. Feel harmony and peace being restored in your body and join the trio of colors arched above your head.

You look down at your feet and notice that there is one ray left—the blue. And inhaling now, you pull this beautiful blue ray in through your feet. And as you do so, an even deeper state of tranquillity comes over you; a heightened sense of relaxation prevails. Blue symbolizes inspiration, creativity, and faith. Blue calms and cools. Let your body respond to these special qualities of the color blue. Relax. Enjoy the feeling of this soothing, cooling color moving throughout your body. If any part of your body feels inflamed or irritated, envision blue light flowing to that area, cooling, calming, and relaxing. Now let the color blue spiral upward throughout your body and filter out the top of your head to complete the rainbow formed above you.

From the tips of your toes to the top of your head, you have funneled the colors of the rainbow throughout your being, and they have done their healing work. Picture yourself now standing in this beautiful lush meadow with a rainbow of colors crowning your head, with thousands of sunbeams glistening about you and with the warm moist earth beneath your feet. How special you feel. How special you are! And from deep within you there rises now a sense, an indisputable knowing, that all is well. *All is truly well.*

Inhale deeply now and then softly exhale. Inhale gently and again feel yourself being slowly swept up. Exhale and again experience being drawn away—away this time from the meadow and back into the present awareness. Breathe softly and evenly, taking leave of the meadow, letting the image of you, the image of the rainbow gradually fade. Bring back with you the feeling of specialness, of well-being and peace. Ah yes, those exquisite feelings of well-being and peace and the knowing that all is truly well. Softly, gently, quietly come back. Inhale deeply and feel your eyelids part. Exhale now and fully open your eyes.

Relaxation Script 2

Peaceful Body, Quiet Mind

And now it is time to relax. Time to become still. Time to journey to that place deep inside you—that place that knows only the stillness, only the peace, and only the calm. This is not a time to be thinking about outer concerns. Let all memories of the activities of your day gently fade away. Let go all thoughts about the past—all anticipation you may have about the future. Just let the past and the future fade into a blur as you focus only on this present moment of stillness and peace. Position yourself comfortably now in a way that allows your body to easily soften and relax. And if it feels right for you, you may gently close your eyes; letting the closing of your eyes softly usher you away from the outside world, and deeper and deeper and deeper into the calm. Gradually become aware of your breathing. Feel the flow of air, first in, then out of your body. Let your inhale come softly and then release gently into the exhale without effort, force, or strain. Breathe evenly, slowly, gently, allowing the rhythmic flow of your breathing to lull you further into the stillness—further into the peace.

Let no outer sounds distract you. Let no outer thoughts disturb you. Should you find any unwanted thoughts trying to interfere with this time of relaxation and peace, just imagine that right in the center of your mind is a tiny whisk broom that slowly sweeps back and forth, and back and forth, and back and forth. At the first sign of any outside thoughts, just imagine this little whisk broom softly sweeping them away. Let this tiny broom sweep your mind, clean your mind, until your mind is totally clear, relaxed, and calm.

Focus once again on your breathing, feeling the gentle movement of your body as you breathe in and breathe out, breathe in and breathe out, breathe in and breathe out. Let your breathing become slower now, slower and slower as you experience your entire being becoming more and more relaxed.

Visualization Script 2

The Rose, Eucalyptus, and Candle

As you continue to relax, slowly bring to mind the image of a beautiful and fragrant rose. See this rose colored in whatever hue is pleasing to you, with its petals softly opened. Try not to force this image, just let it gradually come forth—keeping your body and mind relaxed and still as the details of the rose slowly come into focus and the image becomes clearer and clearer to you.

Concentrate only on the rose, maintaining the calm even flow of your breathing. And as you inhale now, imagine that you can detect just a hint of the rich fragrance of the rose. Release softly into the exhale so as not to disturb its delicate petals. Inhale slowly once again, this time allowing yourself to capture more of the rose fragrance. Exhale evenly and gently so that the rose remains still. Continue breathing in this soft, gentle manner, allowing yourself to really smell the aroma of this beautiful rose. With each successive breath, allow it to become more and more pronounced. Let the fragrance of the rose enfold you, soothe, and comfort you. And feel your body becoming increasingly tranquil and relaxed. Continue to breathe slowly and deliberately. And as you inhale now imagine that you are drawing in rays of fragrant, rose-colored light. Imagine that with each slow, deeply inhaled breath you are drawing in fragrant rose-colored light that flows freely now throughout the whole of your being. Imagine that with every breath you take, your body opens to take in this light. Continue to breathe slowly, gently, and softly. See yourself engulfed in the fragrance of the rose and surrounded by its beautiful light. Breathe evenly, slowly, softly so as not to disturb the petals of the rose. Breathe evenly, slowly, softly, so as not to disturb the fragrant rays of light.

Gradually now, allow the image of the rose and its fragrant light to fade. Let it go. Continue though the smooth, rhythmic flow of your breathing. Breathe deeply in and softly out. Deeply in and softly out. Letting the image of the rose slip away. Breathe deeply in and softly out.

As your breathing gently ebbs and flows, gradually bring to mind now an image of eucalyptus. Begin to form in your mind a picture perhaps of a sprig or a stalk of this fragrant green plant. Again, do not strain in forming this image; just let it come to you in as clear a form as you can easily fashion. Hold this image of eucalyptus before you now, and become mindful once again of your breathing. Inhale slowly and deeply, letting yourself catch just a whiff of the eucalyptus fragrance. Exhale softly and evenly so as not to disturb the beautiful foliage. Continue breathing in this soft, gentle manner, letting yourself capture with each successive breath more and more of the rich aroma of the eucalyptus. Allow the fragrance of the eucalyptus to enfold you, soothe you, comfort you, absorb you. Feel your body tingle with delight. Continue to breathe slowly and deliberately. And as you inhale now, imagine that you are drawing in soft green rays of light from the eucalyptus. Imagine that with each slow, deeply inhaled breath you are drawing in fragrant green rays of light that now flow freely throughout the whole of your being. Imagine every cell, muscle, and fiber of your body opening to take in this beautiful light. Continue to breathe slowly, gently, and evenly. See yourself engulfed in the fragrance of the eucalyptus and surrounded by its soft, green light. Breathe evenly, slowly, and softly, so as not to disturb the plant's beautiful foliage. Breathe evenly, slowly, and softly, so as not to disturb the fragrant rays of light. Allow yourself to take in one last deeply drawn inhale, and, as you exhale, gradually allow the image of the eucalyptus and its fragrant light to fade. Release it and let it flow from your mind as gently as it came. Continue the smooth, rhythmic flow of your breathing. Empty your mind, clear your mind, as once again you breathe deeply in and softly out. Deeply in and softly out. Deeply in and softly out.

Finally now, picture in your mind's eye a beautiful white tapered candle—its flame burning soft and evenly against the darkness. Take a moment and focus on this candle and its even, steady flame. Breathe gently now so as not to disturb the flame. Breathe softly, slowly, and smoothly, lest the slightest shift in your breathing cause the flame to flicker. Allow nothing to distract you from your focus on the flame nor from the calm, even flow of your breathing. As you focus on the candle, you notice that it gives off a beautiful golden light. Imagine, as you inhale now, that you are drawing in rays of golden light from the candle. Inhale slowly and deeply, filling your body with golden rays of light. Exhale softly and evenly, so as not disturb the glowing candle flame. Continue to draw in the light from the candle, as you imagine every fiber of your being warmed and soothed by its radiant glow. Breathe evenly, slowly, softly, so as not to disturb the steady flame of the candle. Breathe evenly, slowly, softly, so as not to disturb the radiant, golden light. Draw in a long, slow, deep breath now, and with your exhale, blow out the flame. You are surrounded by the darkness now, in a state of total calm. Relaxed and at peace, filled with soothing, fragrant memories of the candle, the eucalyptus, and the rose.

And now as this tape comes to a close, you may wish to allow these soothing images to usher you into a deep, relaxed sleep. Or if you like, let them guide you back into the waking world. Whatever feels right for you is okay. Know, however, that these images are always close at hand, for they are right inside of you. And you can always recapture them whenever you take the time to relax.

Visualization Script 3

The Bridge

You are so relaxed. Your whole being is tranquil and still. With your eyelids closed, it's as if someone has turned out all the lights in the house you call your body, and all your muscles, cells, and organs are fast asleep, nestled into a state of calm repose and rest. No matter what may be occurring on the outside, hold this image of your body being totally relaxed and at peace. Pay close attention to your breathing. Breathe slowly, in and out, through your nose. Breathe evenly, slowly, gently. Let your inhale come softly, and then release gently into the exhale. Notice the feelings and sensations as air flows in, and then flows out your body. Feel the gentle rise and fall of your chest as you breathe in and breathe out; breathe in and breathe out; breathe in and breathe out. Let no outer activity distract you; just become lost in the rhythmic flow of your breathing. And with each breath that you take, just feel yourself letting go—holding on to nothing except a wondrous feeling of drifting deeper and deeper into the stillness, further and further into the peace. You are enveloped in such an exquisite state of calm. Your mind is so relaxed, so detached, so still. It's so easy for comforting thoughts and images to pass through. Feel your mind softening, opening, readying to take in the flow of comforting images and visions.

So in your mind's eye, allow to emerge an image of yourself standing on the bank of a body of water—a body of water that you are about to cross. The crossing of this water represents overcoming, getting past or on the other side of whatever challenge, obstacle, or difficulty you are facing in your life now.

However large you see this challenge, that's how large the body of water is. However discomforting or difficult you view this challenge determines how calm or raging the water. With this in mind, take a moment and create your image of this body of water. Is it a stream or a pond? A lake, a river, or an ocean? Is the water still? Is it smooth or choppy? Or perhaps here and there a bit of both? Compose this image based on your own sense of the magnitude of the obstacle or challenge before you.

Now I want you to imagine that a giant log spans the water, connecting where you are standing now to the other side—where you are going. The log is broad and sturdy, and represents the groundwork that has already been laid by your efforts so far to deal with this challenge, and all the help and support you have received. The log, the groundwork, has been laid. You, however, must walk across.

From where you are standing now, imagine that you can see over to the other side. And as you look, imagine that your eyes connect with the very person or persons, goal, purpose, or heart's desire that makes the overcoming of your obstacle so very important. You feel a deep stirring within you now, as you view in the distance that which makes you determined to get through; that which gives you reason, purpose, and drive to overcome. As you look into the distance, who or what do you see? If not a person, place, or thing, perhaps it is a symbol—your symbol of hope, or of faith. Really allow yourself to experience this passionate sense of purpose, this reason to endure, this will to make it, to triumph, to succeed. Hold fast and tenaciously to it. Let it pulsate throughout your entire being.

Empowered by this clarity of purpose, see yourself now mount the log, and begin to cross the water. If you feel the need, fashion a railing in your mind that you can hold onto for security and support as you cross. Your steps are even and sure. At the first sign of fear, hesitation, or doubt, you stop, breathe deeply, relax, and then proceed again. You realize how easy it is to be thrown off balance by allowing your thoughts to run wild, to race ahead of you. And so you curb unproductive thinking, refuse to entertain any thoughts that extend beyond where you are at the present moment, beyond each step that you are taking one by one right now. If any thoughts prove to be persistent, refuse to get out of the way—pretend to gently pluck them from your mind and toss them into the water. Then watch as they slowly drift away.

See yourself continue to walk across the log. You neither look forward now or backward, but focus only on the step you take each moment. Be encouraged in knowing that no matter how small your steps might be, you are at least moving. Speed is of no importance to you, for you have come to know patience well. You are, above all, moving in the right direction—toward your goal, toward well-being, and toward all that really matters to you.

You continue your trek across the log with even greater confidence now—taking one step at a time, looking neither back to the past, nor too far forward into the future. Being grateful for each sign of movement, and maintaining about and within you a sense of calm, relaxation, and peace. You know that these are the keys to your overcoming, the path you must travel to regain harmony, wholeness, and balance in your life.

Without looking ahead now, you sense that you are close to the other side. Twinges of excitement and anticipation come over you. See yourself take one last step, and then feel your feet touch solid ground. You've made it! You hear the sound of applause. Overjoyed, you look up now, and into the eyes of all those near and dear to you—especially those for whom you were determined to make it. You have reached your goal. You have made it through. You have triumphed at last.

You look back now and take one final glance across the water. What a way you have come! That other side seems so far away now. And you realize with great relief that the past is truly behind you. And so you turn and face the future confidently—filled with love, filled with peace, filled with joy.

Inhale deeply now, and then softly exhale. And holding fast to the feelings of triumph, love, peace, and joy, prepare to come back to your waking state. You have opened your mind to take in a beautiful experience, which you can create again and again and again. Softly, gently, quietly, come back, taking as much time as you need to reacquaint yourself with the outside world. And when you are ready, you may open your eyes.

To order these tapes, please see the last page of this book.

About the Author

Harriett L. Sanders Karis, L.C.S.W., currently serves as Manager of Social Services at the Alta Bates Comprehensive Cancer Center in Berkeley. An experienced practitioner, Harriett conducts relaxation and visualization sessions on an ongoing basis for patients with cancer.

Harriett obtained her B.A. and M.S.W. degrees from Howard University in Washington, D.C. She has worked in the health care field for twenty-four years—the last eleven of which have been exclusively in oncology.

Appendix

Drug Names

Generic Name	Brand Name
acyclovir	Zovirax
bisacodyl	Ducolax
cimetidine	Tagamet
cyclosporine A	Sandimmune
dexamethazone	Decadron, Hexadrol
diazepam	Valium
diphenhydramine hydrochloride	Benadryl
diphenoxylate hydrochloride with atropine sulfate	Lomotil
docusate sodium	Colace, D.S.S.
dronabinol	Marinol
famotidine	Pepcid
granisetron	Kytril
lidocaine hydrochloride 2%	Xylocaine
loperamide hydrochloride	Imodium

lorazepam	Ativan
methyl cellulose	Citrucel
metoclopramide	Reglan
nystatin	Mycostatin
omeprazole	Prilosec
ondansetron hydrochloride	Zofran
phenazopyridine hydrochloride	Pyridium
polymyxin B sulfate, bacitracin zinc, and neomycin sulfate	Neosporin
prochlorperazine	Compazine
psyllium hydrophilic mucilloid	Metamucil
ranitidine hydrochloride	Zantac
silver sulfadiazine 1%	Silvadene
trimethobenzamide hydrochloride	Tigan

Index

Note to the reader: Page numbers in italics refer to tables and figures

A

Chemotherapy and Radiation Therapy Relaxation Tapes

Written and narrated by Harriet Sanders, L.C.S.W., these tapes are based on years of experience leading relaxation groups for people dealing with cancer. Ms. Sanders' voice is a gentle alto that creates confidence and a deep sense of serenity.

BODY RELAXED, MIND AT EASE

This tape helps you systematically let go of tension in every part of your body. You learn to breathe with a strong, deeply peaceful rhythm and to use images of calming light and color to replace hot spots of tension. One 42-minute audiocassette.

Item 40 $11.95

PEACEFUL BODY, QUIET MIND

This powerful tape for healing and recovery uses guided imagery, music, and affirmations to instill a state of positive belief in which you expect to get well and your natural healing powers are harnessed as you focus on your goal. One 60-minute audiocassette.

Item 59 $11.95

Other New Harbinger Titles

MIND OVER MALIGNANCY

Studies show that a patient's ability to feel actively involved in the treatment process is one of the most critical aspects of fighting any illness. This book distills years of clinical experience into a step-by-step program that shows you how to cope with self-defeating stress and depression and develop a fighting attitude, control pain and side-effects, get the support you need, and improve your quality of life—and your chances of survival.

Item MALI $12.95

THE DAILY RELAXER

Presents the most effective and popular techniques for learning how to relax—simple, tension-relieving exercises that you can learn in five minutes and practice with positive results right away.

Item DALY Paperback, $12.95

Call **toll-free 1-800-748-6273** to order. Have your Visa or Mastercard number ready. Or send a check for the titles you want to New Harbinger Publications, 5674 Shattuck Avenue, Oakland, CA 94609. Include $3.80 for the first book and 75¢ for each additional book to cover shipping and handling. (California residents please include appropriate sales tax.) Allow four to six weeks for delivery.

Prices subject to change without notice.

Some Other
New Harbinger Titles

The Cyclothymia Workbook, Item 383X, $18.95

The Matrix Repatterning Program for Pain Relief, Item 3910, $18.95

Transforming Stress, Item 397X, $10.95

Eating Mindfully, Item 3503, $13.95

Living with RSDS, Item 3554 $16.95

The Ten Hidden Barriers to Weight Loss, Item 3244 $11.95

The Sjogren's Syndrome Survival Guide, Item 3562 $15.95

Stop Feeling Tired, Item 3139 $14.95

Responsible Drinking, Item 2949 $18.95

The Mitral Valve Prolapse/Dysautonomia Survival Guide,
Item 3031 $14.95

Stop Worrying Abour Your Health, Item 285X $14.95

The Vulvodynia Survival Guide, Item 2914 $15.95

The Multifidus Back Pain Solution, Item 2787 $12.95

Move Your Body, Tone Your Mood, Item 2752 $17.95

The Chronic Illness Workbook, Item 2647 $16.95

Coping with Crohn's Disease, Item 2655 $15.95

The Woman's Book of Sleep, Item 2493 $14.95

The Trigger Point Therapy Workbook, Item 2507 $19.95

Fibromyalgia and Chronic Myofascial Pain Syndrome, second edition,
Item 2388 $19.95

Kill the Craving, Item 237X $18.95

Rosacea, Item 2248 $13.95

Thinking Pregnant, Item 2302 $13.95

Call **toll free, 1-800-748-6273,** or log on to our online bookstore
at **www.newharbinger.com** to order. Have your Visa or Mastercard
number ready. Or send a check for the titles you want to New Harbinger Publications, Inc., 5674 Shattuck Ave., Oakland, CA 94609.
Include $4.50 for the first book and 75¢ for each additional book, to
cover shipping and handling. (California residents please include
appropriate sales tax.) Allow two to five weeks for delivery.

Prices subject to change without notice.